A Textbook of Orthodontics

A Textbook of Orthodontics

T. D. FOSTER

DDS, FDS, DOrth RCS
Emeritus Professor of
Children's Dentistry and Orthodontics,
University of Birmingham;
Honorary Consultant in
Children's Dentistry and Orthodontics,
Central Birmingham
Health Authority (Teaching)

THIRD EDITION

BLACKWELL SCIENTIFIC PUBLICATIONS

OXFORD LONDON

EDINBURGH BOSTON MELBOURNE

To my wife

First published 1975
Second edition 1982
Third edition 1990

Set by Best-Set Typesetter Ltd, Hong Kong
Printed and bound in Great Britain
by William Clowes Limited,
Beccles and London

DISTRIBUTORS

Marston Book Services Ltd
PO Box 87
Oxford OX2 0DT
(*Orders*: Tel: (0865) 791155
         Fax: (0865) 791927
         Telex: 837515)

USA
Year Book Medical Publishers
200 North LaSalle Street
Chicago, Illinois 60601
(*Orders*: Tel: (312) 726−9733)

Canada
The C. V. Mosby Company
5240 Finch Avenue East
Scarborough, Ontario
(*Orders*: Tel: (416) 298−1588)

Australia
Blackwell Scientific Publications
(Australia) Pty Ltd
107 Barry Street
Carlton, Victoria 3053
(*Orders*: Tel: (103) 347−0300)

British Library
Cataloguing in Publication Data

Foster, T. D. (Thomas Donald)
    A textbook of orthodontics. — 3rd ed.
    1. Dentistry. Orthodontics
    I. Title
    617.6′43

ISBN 0-632-02654-5

Contents

Preface to third edition

The science and art of orthodontics continues to receive a vigourous input, both from research and from clinical development. There is a growing emphasis on the quality of treatment results, particularly from the aspect of functional occlusion, and a growing awareness that treatment of the more complex problems requires careful evaluation and sophisticated appliances in skilled hands. Nevertheless, there remains a need for all dentists to understand the background to the natural occlusion and its variations, and to the rationale of orthodontic treatment, and this remains the aim of the book.

In preparing this third edition, once again the relevant literature of the past six years has been reviewed, and there has been a general updating. Most of the older references have been replaced, though reference to some of the 'classic' historical work remains. The sections on occlusion and on cephalometrics have been largely rewritten, and additions and amendments have been made to all sections of the book in accordance with the most recent research findings. A further change has been the inclusion of a list of references at the end of each chapter, where it is felt they may be more useful than at the end of the book.

I am again indebted to my colleagues and my students for their help, both direct and indirect, and particularly to Dr W. P. Rock, Mr R. I. W. Evans, Dr A. P. Howat and Mr S. Weerakone for the provision of illustrations, and to Miss Jennifer Moses for the preparation of the typescript.

Preface to first edition

Orthodontics is a subject which has aroused a good deal of healthy controversy. Much of the knowledge on the subject has been gained from clinical experience, though there is an increasing emphasis on scientific investigation as a background to clinical methods.

The practice of orthodontics needs to be learned clinically, by practical experience, but a knowledge of the theoretical background is essential for successful practice. This book has been written in order to present the background to current orthodontic practice. It is not intended as a recipe book; rather it is hoped that it provides the student with a rational explanation of the aetiology of the occlusion and position of the natural dentition, and of the treatment of occlusal discrepancies.

Orthodontic practice deals very largely with the wide range of normal variation. For this reason, pathological abnormalities have been excluded and variation has been emphasized. In those areas of the subject where there is difference of opinion, an attempt has been made to put forward the various views where these are supported by evidence from published work, and, where possible, to draw some rational line in the light of personal experience.

In producing this book, I am conscious of the help given, both directly and indirectly by my colleagues. I would like to acknowledge the assistance of those who have made available clinical records and who have helped with the preparation of illustrative material. In particular, I wish to thank Mr M. R. Sharland and Mr M. C. Walker for the production of the photographs, and Miss Jennifer Jones for the preparation of the typescript.

1

Postnatal growth of the skull and jaws

Most orthodontic treatment at the present time is carried out during the growth period, between the ages of 10 and 15 years. The occlusion and position of the teeth is also established during the growth period, and changes after growth has finished are of relatively minor degree. It is probable that interference with the occlusion in the early stages of growth, for example by extraction of teeth, produces some alteration in occlusal development. Furthermore, patterns of growth of the jaws and development of the occlusion, which vary between individuals, may have a bearing on the need for orthodontic treatment and the timing and type of treatment prescribed.

For these reasons a knowledge of growth of the skull and jaws and of occlusal development should be of importance in orthodontic practice. Although at present much orthodontic treatment is carried out on the basis of a snapshot picture of the occlusion, without knowledge of previous growth, there is an increasing awareness that a knowledge of previous growth changes may be important in planning treatment, and that the timing of treatment in relation to growth may facilitate the progress of such treatment.

There are many growth studies in progress in various parts of the world which have particular emphasis on dental occlusion. There is also much research on growth of the skull and jaws in more general terms. In spite of this, such growth is far from being completely understood, particularly because a great deal of variation exists in the detail of growth changes. This variation makes it difficult to formulate general rules about growth changes, except in very broad terms.

In this chapter it is proposed to outline the present knowledge on postnatal skull and jaw growth, asking the questions *when*, *where*, *how* and *why* does growth proceed.

The skull and jaws at birth

At birth, the skull is far from being merely a small version of the adult skull. There are differences in shape, in proportion of the face and the cranium and in the degree of development and fusion of the individual bones. Some bones, which in the adult are single bones, are still in separate constituent parts at birth. Other bones, which in the adult are closely joined to their neighbours at sutures, are, at birth, widely separated from neighbouring bones. Bones which have developed from cartilage, mainly those at the base of the skull, still have a cartilaginous element actively growing. Bones which have developed from membrane, mainly those of the calvarium and face, still have wide membranous areas at their margins actively forming bone. The main features of the skull at birth can be summarized as follows (Figs. 1.1, 1.2, 1.3).

Bones in separate component parts

1 At the base of the skull the sphenoid bone is in three parts, the central body with its two lesser wings, and on each side the greater wing and its attached pterygoid process.
2 The occipital bone is in two parts, the condylar part which carries the occipital condyles, and the squamous part, much of which has developed from membrane and forms part of the calvarium.
3 The temporal bone on each side is in two parts, the petromastoid component which has developed from the cartilaginous neurocranium,

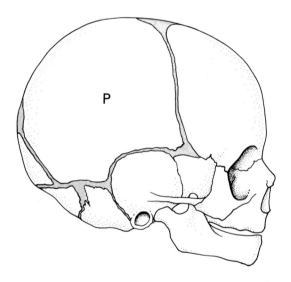

Fig. 1.1. Side view of the skull at birth, showing the wide separation of the cranial bones and the fontanelles at the corners of the parietal bone (P). The main components of the occipital bone are still ununited.

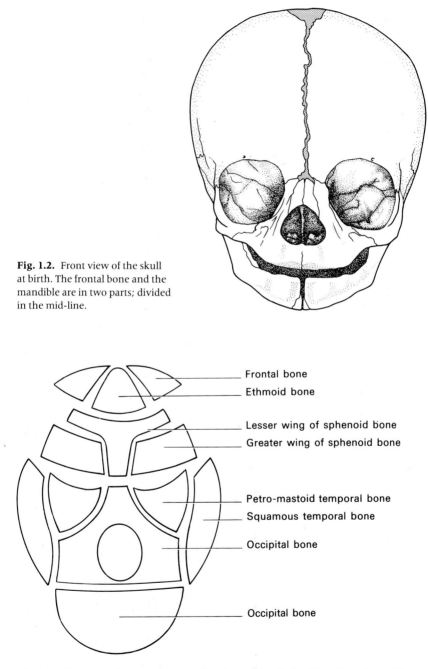

Fig. 1.2. Front view of the skull at birth. The frontal bone and the mandible are in two parts; divided in the mid-line.

Frontal bone
Ethmoid bone

Lesser wing of sphenoid bone
Greater wing of sphenoid bone

Petro-mastoid temporal bone
Squamous temporal bone

Occipital bone

Occipital bone

Fig. 1.3. Diagrammatic representation of the base of the skull at birth. The sphenoid bone is in three component parts, the temporal bones in two parts and the occipital bone in two parts.

and the squamous component which has developed from the membranous neurocranium.

4 The frontal bone and the mandible, which will eventually become single bones, are each in two parts at birth, the parts being separated in the mid-sagittal plane.

Bones widely separated from neighbouring bones

In general, the sutures of the skull are wider at birth than in the adult, being areas of active bone formation. This separation is particularly noticeable at the four corners of the parietal bone where the areas of membrane between the parietal bone and neighbouring bones form the six fontanelles. These are the anterior and posterior fontanelles in the mid-sagittal plane where the parietal bones meet the frontal and occipital bones respectively, and the antero-lateral and postero-lateral fontanelles on each side, at the junction of parietal, sphenoid and frontal bones and parietal, temporal and occipital bones respectively.

The sphenoid and occipital bones, which eventually will become fused at the base of the skull, are still separated at birth by a cartilaginous area, the spheno-occipital synchondrosis.

Relative sizes of the face and the cranium

The relationship in size between the face and the cranium is noticeably different at birth from that in the adult. The cranium, or more properly the neurocranium, has grown rapidly in the prenatal period, accommodating the rapidly developing brain. The face, or viscerocranium, has developed less towards its adult size than has the cranium, with the result that at birth the face appears small in the vertical dimension in relation to the total size of the head when compared with the proportions in the adult (Fig. 1.4). The main reasons for this lie in the form of the maxilla and mandible. These bones, which form the main contribution to the vertical dimension of the face, are relatively small at birth. The maxillary antrum is little more than a flat space, compared with its much greater vertical depth in the adult (Fig. 1.5). The mandible is relatively straight, with a more obtuse gonial angle than in the adult. In both bones there are no erupted teeth, and consequently little vertical development of alveolar bone. The articular fossae for the mandible on the temporal bones are relatively flat, giving possibility for a wide range of mandibular movement.

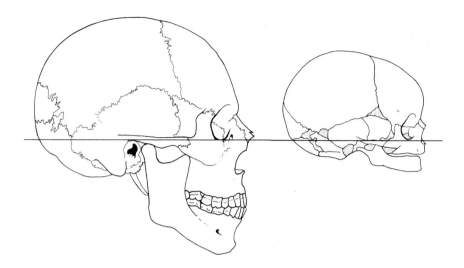

Fig. 1.4. Relative sizes of face and cranium at birth and in adult life. At birth the cranium forms a much larger proportion of the head than in the adult.

From this condition at birth, the head grows to its adult size and proportions. When, where, how and why does it grow?

Rates of growth from birth to adult

At birth, the head forms about one quarter of the total height of the body. In the adult the head forms about one eighth of total body height. Therefore between birth and maturity the body must grow faster, in proportion to size, than the head. In most individuals the general rate of body growth follows a pattern, although there is variation in the detailed timing of the different phases of this pattern. In infancy, growth proceeds at a relatively high rate, slowing progressively during child-hood to reach a minimum rate in the prepuberal period. There is then an increase in growth rate during puberty and finally a marked slowing in growth rate to maturity (Fig. 1.6). The age at which these phases of growth begin and end varies between individuals and between the sexes.

While the total growth of the head from birth to maturity is proportionately less than that of the rest of the body, the head itself does not grow at a constant rate. the two main components of the head, that is the cranium and the face, differ in their relative proportion at birth and at maturity, and therefore they must grow at differing rates, neither of which is constant. The two components can be considered separately.

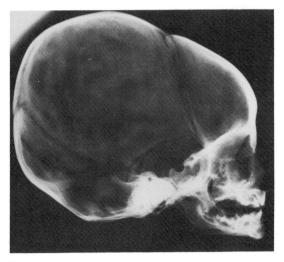

a

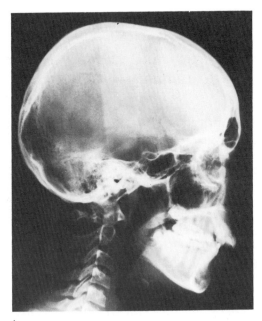

b

Fig. 1.5. Radiographs of the skull (a) at birth; and (b) in adult life, showing the increase in size of the maxillary antrum.

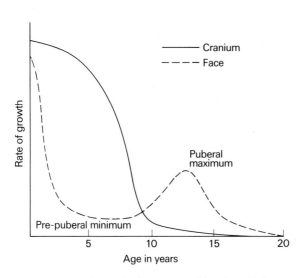

Fig. 1.6. Rates of growth of cranium and face from birth to maturity in boys.

Growth rate of the cranium

The cranium, which has grown rapidly before birth, continues to grow rapidly up to about 1 year of age, accommodating the brain, which at this stage is developing to provide an enormous increase in physical and mental activity. Thereafter the growth rate decreases, and by about 7 years of age the cranium has reached some 90% of its final volume (Fig. 1.7). There is then a slow increase in size to maturity (Fig. 1.6).

The growth rate of the eyes, and consequently of the eye sockets, follows a similar pattern.

Thus the infant, by comparison with the adult, appears to have a small face, with large eyes, large cranium and retrusive nose.

Growth rate of the face

The growth rate of the face, which is highest at birth, falls sharply and reaches a prepuberal minimum level, some 2 years earlier in girls than in boys. Growth rate then increases to a peak at puberty, declining again and tailing off until growth ceases in late teenage (Fig. 1.6). Facial growth is normally associated with eruption of the primary dentition between 1 and 3 years of age and of the permanent dentition between 6 and 14 years of age, when the erupting teeth and developing alveolar

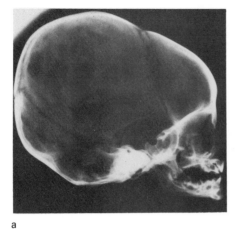

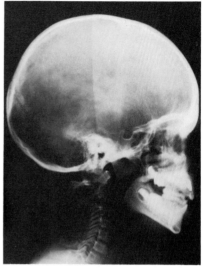

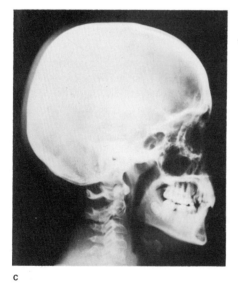

Fig. 1.7. Radiographs of the skull at (a) birth; (b) 6 years; and (c) maturity. At 6 years the cranium has almost reached adult size, but the face is noticeably smaller than in the adult.

process add to the total size of the jaws. Studies of dental arch growth by Van der Linden (1983) and others have suggested that increase in size of the dental arches is particularly associated with tooth eruption. During the period of the established primary dentition there is little change in the dimensions of the dental arches and thus in the length and breadth of the tooth bearing parts of the jaws. However, the serial studies of growth of the head carried out by Brodie (1941) have shown that during the same period the total length and height of the jaws increases and the face is progressively positioned downward and forward in relation to the cranium, a process known as translation.

It would appear that facial growth rate follows roughly the same pattern as the rate of body growth. The work of Lewis *et al.* (1985) has shown that forward and downward growth of both maxilla and mandible follow this pattern, and the period of maximum puberal growth of the jaws is a few months later than that of body height. Hägg and Pancherz (1983) have found a close relationship between maximum puberal growth in standing height and maximum condylar growth. It is also suggested that mandibular growth continues on average about 2 years longer than maxillary growth (Lewis & Roche 1988). This difference in growth between the two jaws may be important in orthodontic treatment planning, as also may individual differences in the rates of growth at various ages, particularly the age of the puberal growth spurt.

Mechanisms of growth and areas of growth

While the possibilites for how the skull grows can be fairly clearly elicited, the question of where growth actually takes place during various phases of the growth period is not so well understood.

Bone, unlike most other tissues, cannot grow simply by interstitial division of its living cells to give increasing size. There are three main mechanisms of bone growth, each of which plays its part in the growth of the skull and jaws.

1 Cartilaginous growth—the growth of cartilage by cell division, with progressive conversion to bone by ossification.

2 Sutural growth—the apposition of bone in the area of the sutures between adjacent bones.

3 Periosteal and endosteal growth—the apposition of bone under the periosteal membrane and at the surfaces of the cancellous spaces within the bone.

Cartilaginous growth

The areas of the skull where cartilaginous growth is possible are mainly at the base of the skull, in the area of the nasal septum and at the head of the mandibular condyle (Fig. 1.8). Growth of cartilage at the spheno-occipital synchondrosis would increase the antero-posterior dimension

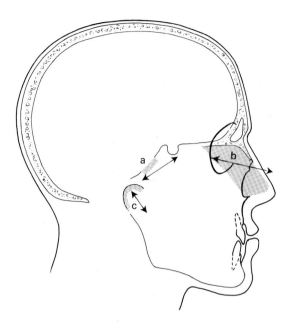

Fig. 1.8. Areas of cartilaginous growth in the head. (a) Spheno-occipital synchondrosis; (b) nasal septum; (c) mandibular condyle.

of the skull base. Growth of the nasal septal cartilage would bring the nose forward from its original position under the front of the cranium. Growth of the mandibular condylar cartilage would increase the total length and height of the mandible. It seems likely that all these areas of cartilage growth play their part in the total growth of the head, at least in the early years. Whether they are active after puberty remains in some doubt.

Sutural growth

The bony sutures of the head are such that sutural growth would be capable of increasing the size of the head in all dimensions (Fig. 1.9). It has been suggested that the sutures which separate the face from the cranium are aligned so that growth at these sutures would move the face in a forward and downward direction in relation to the cranium, and longitudinal studies such as that of Brodie (1941) have shown that this is indeed the general direction of relative growth. However, there is no strong evidence that such directional growth is in fact brought about by growth at the sutures, and Remmelink (1988) has reported that the retro-maxillary sutural surfaces in the human skull are mainly sagittally

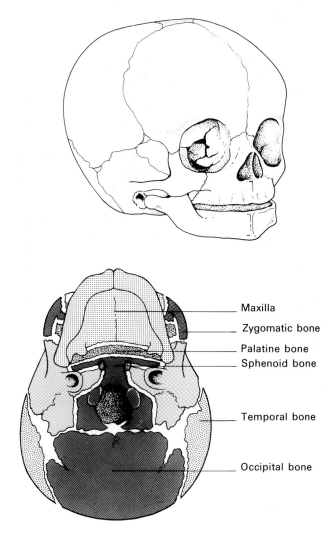

Fig. 1.9. Suture systems of the head.

orientated. In the very early years, when the bones of the skull are widely separated from each other, sutural growth is active in bringing the bones into close proximity. When the sutures have formed, some sutural growth must take place concomitant with enlargement of the bone, if such enlargement is accompanied by increase in total length of the suture. Therefore sutural growth must be active at the time of main enlargement of the cranium, that is up to 6 or 7 years of age, though the importance of such growth thereafter is in some doubt.

Periosteal and endosteal growth

The apposition of bone on the periosteal surfaces would obviously enlarge the head in all dimensions. It would also cause the bones to be excessively thickened and therefore concomitant resorption of bone is necessary in order to obtain the appropriate thickness and strength. However, periosteal growth is not simply a matter of addition of bone to the outer surface and resorption of bone from the inner surface. Extensive remodelling of bones takes place, which often involves resorption of bone from the outer surface and apposition of bone on the inner surface. Endosteal resorption and addition of bone from within the cancellous spaces is also necessary to maintain the appropriate thickness of the cortical layer of bone.

It is probable that periosteal and endosteal growth plays an important part in the growth of the head. The vital staining experiments of Brash (1924) have shown that the development of the alveolar processes of the jaws is brought about by apposition and remodelling of this type. It is generally thought that this method of growth is the most active type of growth in the skull and jaws after the first few years of life, when cartilaginous and sutural growth slows.

In the light of knowledge of the mechanisms by which the bony elements of the head can be enlarged, the following appears to be the current state of knowledge and belief as to how growth actually occurs, although it must be emphasized that there is difference of opinion and that knowledge is far from complete.

THE SKULL BASE

All three mechanisms of bone growth play their parts in enlargement of the cranial base. Cartilaginous growth, particularly at the spheno-occipital synchondrosis, can cause antero-posterior expansion. According to Powell and Brodie (1964) this synchondrosis does not ossify until 12−16 years of age, and it may therefore be producing active growth to the age of puberty. Sutural growth at the sutures bordering the sphenoid and occipital bones allows lateral growth of the cranial base and is probably active up to 6 or 7 years of age. Periosteal and endosteal growth provides both increase in size and alteration in shape of the bones of the cranial base.

THE CRANIAL VAULT

Most of the growth of the cranial vault is complete by about 7 years of age. Both sutural growth and periosteal and endosteal growth play their parts. Sutural growth is particularly active in the early years, when the bones, original widely separated at birth, grow together. The suture in the mid-line between the frontal bones is normally ossified by the eighth year of life and it seems unlikely that sutural growth in the cranial vault is active after this age. Periosteal and endosteal growth, as well as increasing the overall size and thickness of the bones, alters their form. For example, the parietal bones, which are relatively flat at birth, become markedly concave by the end of the growth period.

THE FACIAL SKELETON

The development of the face generally follows the pattern of growth rate of the rest of the body, possibly lagging slightly behind in time.

The nasal portion of the upper part of the facial skeleton develops forward in response to cartilaginous growth of the nasal septum, bringing the nose out as a protruberance on the face rather than as the largely intra-facial feature of the infant (Fig. 1.10).

The face develops in a forward and downward direction in relation

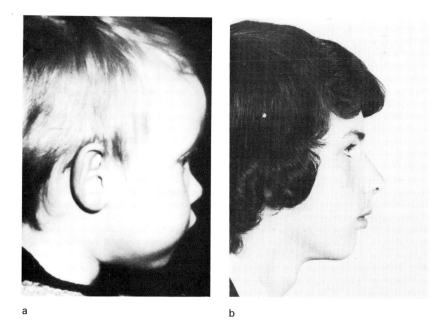

a   b

Fig. 1.10. Growth of the nasal septum changes the nose from the intra-facial feature of the infant to the protruberant feature of the adult face.

to the cranium. Sutural growth in the retrofacial area, i.e. the sutures dividing the maxilla from the retrofacial bones, and the retrofacial bones from the base of the skull (Fig. 1.9) would allow this. Similarly, mid-line suture growth would allow expansion of the maxilla. Björk and Skeiller (1977), using implant studies, have confirmed that both lowering and widening of the maxilla occurs throughout the growth period, and suggest that this is associated with sutural growth.

Periosteal and endosteal growth is undoubtedly very important in facial growth. Postnatal growth in height, breadth and length of the maxilla is largely brought about by periosteal and endosteal growth, which forms the alveolar processes at the teeth erupt, and causes the increase in size of the maxillary antrum by concomitant resorption and remodelling.

The mandible grows by cartilaginous and periosteal and endosteal growth. Two areas of cartilage exist, one at the mandibular symphysis and the other forming a cap on the head of each mandibular condyle. These cartilages are not remnants of Meckel's cartilage, which formed the embryonic precursor of the mandible, but are secondary cartilages which develop after Meckel's cartilage is largely replaced by intramembranous ossification. The symphysial cartilage grows and produces bone during the first year of life, but becomes ossified by the end of the first year. The role of the condylar cartilage in mandibular growth is the subject of some controversy. It has previously been thought that the condylar cartilage is analogous to an epiphyseal cartilage, but Ronning and Koski (1969) have suggested that it is primarily associated with the articulatory function of the condyle. Meikle (1973a, 1973b) has shown that the cellular layer covering the condyle is capable of forming bone or cartilage, the latter being formed when normal articulatory function is present. Thus the condylar cartilage itself may not be a specific growth centre, but it is widely thought that bone growth in the condylar region is necessary for normal mandibular size and form.

Periosteal and endosteal growth are important in the growth of the mandible. The alveolar process develops by this means, and a large amount of surface apposition and remodelling takes place between birth and maturity. The classic studies of mandibular growth by Hunter (1771), Humphrey (1864), Brash (1924) and others have suggested that, during growth, bone is added to the posterior surface and resorbed from the anterior surface of the mandibular ramus, which also tends to increase the length of the mandibular body (Fig. 1.11). Furthermore, addition and resorption of bone on the complex multidirectional surfaces of the mandible serve to produce growth in all dimensions.

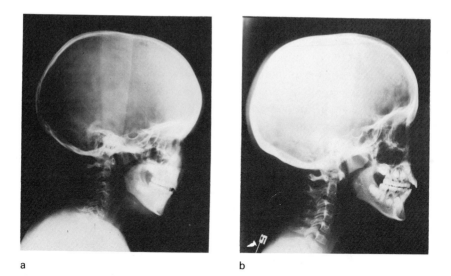

a   b

Fig. 1.11. Radiographs of the skull (a) at 4 years and (b) at 8 years of age showing how resorption of bone at the anterior surface of the mandibular ramus makes space for the eruption of the permanent molar teeth.

Björk and Skeiller (1977, 1983) have pointed out that, during the growth period, both maxilla and mandible undergo rotation relative to the anterior cranial base when viewed from the lateral aspect. This rotation is variable both in degree and in direction, with forward and upward rotation being the most common, but with rotation in both directions sometimes occurring in an individual during the growth period. From studies of growth using metallic implants in the jaws, they have identified stable structures within the jaws which retain their relationships with each other during growth. They have postulated that the *total rotation* of the mandible is the rotation of the mandible corpus as identified by the stable structures, relative to the anterior cranial base. The *matrix rotation* is the rotation of the mandible as a whole, including the periostial appositional elements and the *intra-matrix rotation* is the difference between total and matrix rotation, representing only the periostal remodelling of the jaw. Solow and Houston (1988) have suggested the terms *true rotation*, *apparent rotation*, and *angular re-modelling* respectively as alternatives to those of Björk and Skeiller (1977, 1983). The significance of growth rotations is that they can alter jaw relationships during growth, especially in the vertical plane. However, since they vary considerably between individuals, the accuracy of their prediction is in doubt.

The reasons for growth of the head

The rates, sites and mechanisms of bone growth in the head have been the subject of considerable study, and, as has been mentioned, knowledge is still incomplete, particularly regarding the various types of growth which are important at different stages. There is even less knowledge, and more difference of opinion, on the question of why the bones of the head grow to their final size and form. In past decades function was thought to be important in determining form, and it was held that the bones of the face in particular could be influenced in their growth by their function, particularly dietary and respiratory function. More recently it has been felt that the bones have an inherent potential to achieve their predetermined size and form, provided that pathological features do not intervene, and that function plays little part. The functional aspect of growth has now come to the fore again in a somewhat different light, particularly with the theories of Moss (1968). Moss's theory of the functional matrix postulates that the bones of the head grow in response to the function of two types of matrix, the periosteal matrix, which includes the facial muscles and the teeth, and the capsular matrix, which includes the neural mass and the functional spaces of the mouth, nose and pharynx. The periosteal matrix is responsible for altering the size and shape of the bones, while the capsular matrix alters spatial relationships between various parts of the head. He further postulates that it is the matrix which has the inherent potential for development, rather than the bones themselves.

In considering the reasons for growth of the head, it would be unrealistic to regard the bones independently from their function. The function of the craniofacial skeleton is to provide support and protection for the major seat of central nervous activity, as well as for four of the five special senses, and for part of the activities of respiration and communication. In addition it provides in part the means of ingestion of food and the beginning of the digestive process. The bones are therefore intimately concerned with the brain, the muscles, the teeth and the special sense organs, and it would be reasonable to assume that growth and development of all these items is interdependent. Inheritance certainly plays a large part, as is seen from studies of identical twins, though it seems that there is room for some variation in growth even with the same genetic structure.

Various studies have suggested that normal growth of the cranium and the orbit is in response to growth of the brain and the eye and if this is so it may be reasonable to suppose that normal growth of the lower facial skeleton is in response to growth of the tongue, dentition and the facial and masticatory muscles. Latham and Scott (1970) have postulated that there is a multiple assurance principle involved in facial growth, that is that several systems are involved in producing growth, and if one system fails others continue to produce growth. It must be emphasized that there is a certain independence of growth even of intimately connected parts of the head if pathological conditions intervene. For example, the cellular tissue at the head of the mandibular condyle is particularly vulnerable to damage by trauma or infection. If this tissue is damaged, this has an effect on the growth of the mandible, but there is little or no effect on the growth of the masticatory muscles or on their bony attachments to the jaws. The effect on growth seems to be confined to that growth contributed in the condylar cartilage area, that is, growth in length and height of the mandible, and even appositional bone growth does not seem to be affected.

There have been many studies of the effects of pathological conditions on facial growth. However, while it is desirable to understand normal growth in order to interpret pathological changes, it is probably much less realistic to attempt to understand normal growth from a study of pathological conditions. In the light of present knowledge it would seem reasonable to believe that normal growth of the head depends on the complex interrelationship of growth of all the components, including the function of the muscular components, with a large genetic element involved in both rates and timing of growth and in determination of final size and form.

Normal variation

Variation exists between normal individuals both in growth and in the final form and size of the head, quite apart from the effect of any pathological conditions. Indeed, the main bulk of orthodontic treatment deals with the amendment of normal variation. Variation in growth is largely variation in the rates and amount of growth at different ages. Perhaps the best example of this is the variation in the timing of the puberal growth spurt. There is a general sex difference in the age at the puberal growth spurt, with females tending to exhibit puberal growth some 2 years earlier than males. There are also individual differences. In a study of mandibular growth in girls, Tofani (1972) found that the age of maximum puberal growth in length ranged from 11 to 13 years, and the duration of the total growth spurt ranged from 2½ to 3 years. Thus prediction of the final dimensions of the jaws in a growing child, or the age at which those dimensions will be attained is difficult, although some work has been done on such prediction.

Variation in the final form and size of the head falls into two broad categories, racial variation and individual variation.

RACIAL VARIATION

The different ethnic groups of mankind have a tendency to exhibit certain broad patterns of form of the skull and jaws, although such patterns are often overshadowed by individual variation. In particular the gnathic index, that is the proportion of dental alveolar bone length to the length of basal bone of the jaws, expressed as a percentage, tends to vary between certain ethnic groups. Thus the mongoloid races tend to be mesognathic, having the alveolar length somewhat less than the basal length, and the negroid races tend to be prognathic, having alveolar length somewhat greater than basal length (Fig. 1.12). However, as previously mentioned, there is much individual variation within ethnic groups, possibly as a result of population mixture, and racial variation can only be described in very broad terms.

INDIVIDUAL VARIATION

Variation in skull and jaw size and form between individuals is so common and so well known that it hardly needs description. It seems

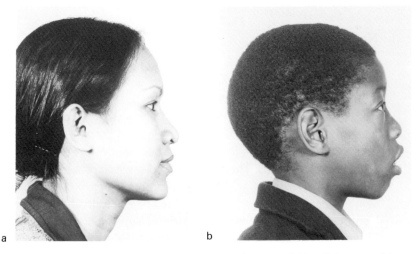

a   b

Fig. 1.12. Racial variation in jaw form. (a) Mesognathic mongoloid, and (b) prognathic negroid profiles.

likely that such variation is largely genetically determined, and this view is supported by twin studies (Fig. 1.13). Several authors have reported the strong genetic influence in the development of facial and jaw form and relationships (Nakasima *et al.* 1982; Lobb 1987; Lundström & McWilliam 1987). Mixtures of populations, such as have been possible to a much greater degree in more recent times, would tend to increase such variation. Individual variation is so complex that it is hardly realistic to describe ideals or norms for all the parameters of skull and jaw size and form. It is more realistic to say that 'normal' indicates anything not involving pathological change, and to regard all non-pathological features as existing within the wide range of normal variation.

Summary

The skull and jaws at birth

1 Some bones are in separate component parts:
  - Sphenoid.
  - Occipital.
  - Temporal.
  - Frontal.
  - Mandible.

2 Most bones are widely separated from neighbouring bones.

3 Fontanelles at the corners of the parietal bone:
  - Antero-lateral (2).
  - Postero-lateral (2).
  - Anterior.
  - Posterior.

4 The face is relatively small in relation to the cranium.
  - Small jaws.
  - Little development of alveolar processes and teeth.
  - Maxillary antrum small.
  - Nose intra-facial.

Rates of growth—birth to adult

1 The head grows slower than the body.

2 The cranium grows slower than the face.

3 Cranial growth is rapid up to 1 year, slowing to reach 90% of final size by 7 years.

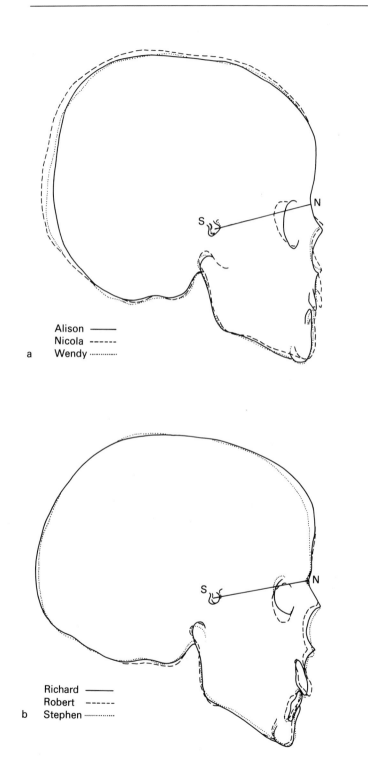

Alison ——
Nicola -----
a   Wendy ··········

Richard ——
Robert -----
b   Stephen ··········

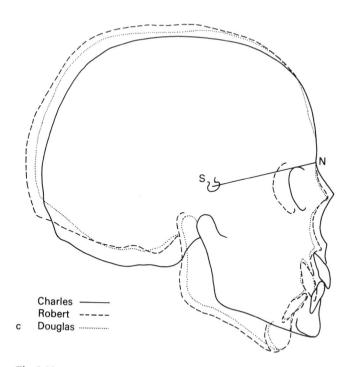

Charles ────
Robert ─ ─ ─ ─
c   Douglas ··············

Fig. 1.13. Tracings of superimposed radiographs of (a) and (b) monozygotic, and (c) dizygotic triplets. The monozygotic triplets show very similar outlines of skull and jaw form, as do the monozygotic pair of the dizygotic triplets. The third member of the dizygotic triplets, who is genetically different, shows a markedly different skull and jaw outline.

4   Facial growth follows the general body growth curve. Rapid early growth diminishes to prepuberal minimum. Puberal growth spurt. Slow final growth to maturity.

Mechanisms and areas of growth

1   Cartilaginous growth. This occurs at the base of skull and nasal septum—possibly until 12 to 16 years of age. Mandibular condyle growth is important, but doubt exists regarding the role of the condylar cartilage.

2   Sutural growth. This is important in the early years when cranial bones are enlarging. There is some doubt regarding importance after 6–7 years of age.

3   Periosteal and endosteal growth. This enlarges the head in all dimensions. It is responsible for growth and remodelling by apposition and resorption of bone.

- In the cranium—most important up to 6 or 7 years of age.
- In the face—important throughout the growth period.
- Responsible for the development of the alveolar processes of the jaws, concomitant with tooth eruption.

Reasons for growth

1 Different theories have been held favouring function and inheritance as the main factor in facial growth.
2 Probably an interdependence of growth of all the components of the head.
3 Some independence of growth is exhibited in certain pathological conditions.
4 Growth in normal development is largely genetically determined.

Normal variation

1 Variation in growth rate.
2 Variation in final size, form and relationships.
3 Sex differences in size and in growth rate.
4 Racial variation—sometimes masked by individual variation.
5 Individual variation—probably largely genetically determined.

References

Björk, A. & Skieller, V. (1977) Growth of the maxilla in three dimensions as revealed radiographically by the implant method. *Br J Orthod*, **4**, 53−64.

Björk, A. & Skeiller, V. (1983) Normal and abnormal growth of the mandible: a synthesis of longitudinal cephalometric implant studies over a period of 25 years. *Eur J Orthod*, **5**, 1−46.

Brash, J. C. (1924) The growth of the jaws and palate. In *The Growth of the Jaws in Health and Disease*. London, Dental Board of the United Kingdom.

Brodie, A. G. (1941) Growth patterns of the human head from the third month to the eighth year of life. *Am J Anat*, **68**, 209−262.

Hägg, U. & Pancherz, H. (1988) Dentofacial orthopaedics in relation to chronological age, growth period and skeletal development. *Eur J Orthod*, **10**, 169−176.

Humphrey, G. M. (1864) On the growth of the jaws. *Trans Cambridge Philosophical Soc.*

Hunter, J. (1771) *The Natural History of the Human Teeth*. London, Johnson.

Latham, R. A. & Scott, J. H. (1970) A newly postulated factor in the early growth of the human middle face, and the theory of multiple assurance. *Arch Oral Biol*, **15**, 1097−1100.

Lewis, A. B. & Roche, A. F. (1988) Late growth changes in the craniofacial skeleton. *Angle Orthod*, **58**, 127−135.

Lewis, A. B., Roche, A. F. & Wagner, B. (1985) Pubertal growth spurts in cranial base and mandible. *Angle Orthod*, **55**, 17–30.

Lobb, W. K. (1987) Craniofacial morphology and occlusal variation in monozygous and dizygous twins. *Angle Orthod*, **57**, 219–233.

Lundström, A. & McWilliam, J. S. (1987) A comparision of vertical and horizontal cephalometric variables with regard to hereditability. *Eur J Orthod*, **9**, 104–108.

Meikle, M. C. (1973a) The role of the condyle in the postnatal growth of the mandible. *Am J Orthod*, **64**, 50–62.

Meikle, M. C. (1973b) In vivo transplantation of the mandibular joint of the rat; an autoradiographic investigation into cellular changes at the condyles. *Arch Oral Biol,* **18**, 1011–1020.

Moss, M. L. (1968) The primacy of functional matrices in orofacial growth. *Dent Practit*, **19**, 65–73.

Nakasima, A., Ichinose, M., Nakata, S. & Takahama, Y. (1982) Hereditary factors in the craniofacial morphology of Angle's Class II and Class III malocclusions. *Am J Orthod*, **82**, 150–156.

Powell, T. V. & Brodie, A. G. (1964) Closure of the spheno-occipital synchondrosis. *Anat Rec*, **147**, 15–23.

Remmelink, H. J. (1988) Orientation of maxillary sutural surfaces. *Eur J Orthod*, **10** 223–226.

Ronning, O. & Koski, K. (1969) The effect of the articular disc on the growth of condylar cartilage transplants. *Eur Orthod Soc Trans,* pp. 99–108.

Solow, B. & Houston, W. J. B. (1988) Mandibular rotations: concepts and terminology. *Eur J Orthod*, **10**, 177–179.

Tofani, M. I. (1972) Mandibular growth at puberty. *Am J Orthod*, **62**, 176–195.

Van der Linden, P. F. G. M. (1983) *Development of the Dentition*. Chicago, Quintessence Publishing Co.

2

The occlusion of the teeth

The main functions of the oral cavity can be listed as follows.

1 *The ingestion and digestion of food*

- Suckling
- Chewing
- Swallowing
- Taste

2 *The provision of an accessory airway*

This acts as an adjunct to the nasal airway under certain conditions, e.g. physical stress, respiratory disease.

3 *As part of the process of speech and expression*

Of these functions, the position and occlusion of the teeth plays an important part in chewing and swallowing and probably also in speech. Faulty occlusion may also lead to other problems, for example, disease of the periodontal tissues or disorders of temporo-mandibular joint function.

The occlusion of the teeth can be considered under two headings:

1 *Static occlusion* refers to any position in which the upper and lower teeth come together in contact.

2 *Functional occlusion* refers to the functional movement of the mandible and thus the lower dentition in contact with the upper dentition.

There can be many positions of static occlusion and many aspects of functional occlusion in an individual, and although, as will be seen later, the term 'occlusion' in orthodontics is often applied to one particular static position, there is a growing awareness of the importance of correct functional occlusion.

The broad patterns of tooth position are governed by the size, form and relationship of the jaws and the muscles of the lips, cheeks and tongue. The teeth develop in the jaws, and as they erupt into the oral cavity they are guided into position by the facial and tongue muscles, ideally with the tongue on the inside of the dental arches and the lips and cheeks forming the peripheral guiding forces (Fig. 2.1). The fine detail of tooth position is probably determined ideally by the resting and functioning positions of the mandible, although the situation can be reversed, and faulty tooth position can influence mandibular function, as will be seen. Mandibular positions and movements are obviously fundamental to dental occlusion and though they exhibit an infinite variation, the main features can be described. There is, unfortunately, little general agreement on the terminology regarding occlusion and mandibular position. It is hoped that the following description will give a rational explanation, although differences in terminology still exist.

Mandibular positions

Non-occlusal positions of the mandible

1 Rest position

The position of the mandible at rest, sometimes called the endogenous postural position is the position when all the muscles controlling

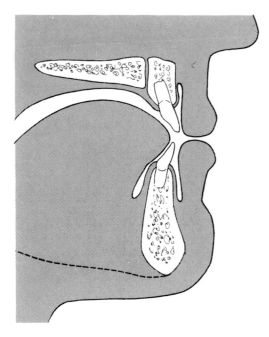

Fig. 2.1. The erupting teeth are guided into position by the muscular activity of the lips, cheeks and tongue.

mandibular position are in a relaxed posture. It is thought to be maintained by a reflex mechanism initiated by the stretch receptors in the masticatory muscles, particularly the temporal muscles. The rest position in most cases is such that there is a space of a few millimetres between the upper and lower teeth. This space is known as the *free-way space*, or *interocclusal clearance*.

Although the rest position of the mandible has been considered to be constant for any individual, there are variations both in the short-term and in the long-term. Everyday variation in the rest position is seen with variation in head posture. Thus if the head is tilted back the interocclusal clearance is increased, if tilted forward the interocclusal clearance is decreased. Long-term variation is related to loss of teeth and possibly to ageing and alteration in muscle tone.

2   Adaptive postural positions

Although in most individuals the mandible takes up the normal rest position, in some a different position is habitually taken up at rest. Such a position can be regarded as an adaptive postural position, because it is a subconscious response to an underlying need. The two main causes for adaptive postural positions are:

(a) To maintain an anterior oral seal. Normal quiet respiration is via the nasal airway. This necessitates the closure of the oral airway, which is

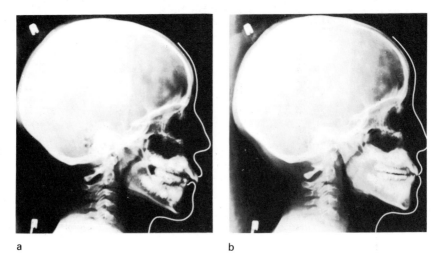

a   b

Fig. 2.2. If the mandible is in a post-normal relationship to the maxilla (a) it may be necessary to adopt a forward posture of the mandible in order to obtain an anterior oral seal (b).

usually achieved by means of a posterior oral seal, with the soft palate touching the tongue, and an anterior oral seal, with the lips in contact or the tongue touching the anterior teeth. In some people the mandible develops in an excessively postnormal relationship to the maxilla and to achieve an anterior oral seal it is necessary to adopt a forward postural position of the mandible (Fig. 2.2).

(b) To achieve oral respiration. If nasal respiration is insufficient it is necessary to substitute or supplement with oral respiration. This is usually the result of restriction in the nasal airway through chronic infection, although of course oral respiration is normal during physical exercise and during speech. For oral respiration it is necessary to adopt an altered postural position of the mandible, with the mandible lowered and an excessive inter-occlusal clearance (see Fig. 2.3).

Occlusal positions of the mandible (static occlusion)

The positions of the mandible with the teeth in occlusal contact are, of course, infinitely variable. Two main positions can be described.

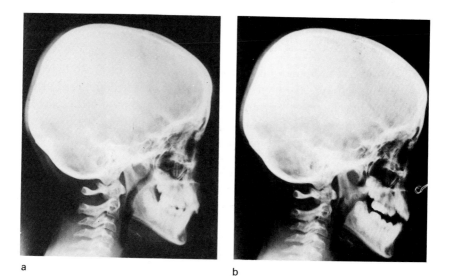

a   b

Fig. 2.3. (a) Nasal respiration. The soft palate is in contact with the tongue, forming a posterior oral seal. (b) Oral respiration. The mandible is lowered and the soft palate elevated to maintain an oral airway.

*1   Retruded contact position (*centric relation)

The terminal position of the automatic path of mandibular movement from rest to occlusion which has not been deviated by tooth contact or abnormal muscle action. The mandibular condyles are normally in their most posterior position in the condylar fossae, though not forcefully retruded.

*2   Intercuspal position (*centric occlusion)

The position of maximum intercuspation of the upper and lower teeth. This definition cannot be applied to every individual, because in some circumstances, as in the later stages of the primary dentition, attrition has reduced the cusps of the teeth so that the occlusal surfaces are relatively flat.

In the majority of people these two occlusal positions of the mandible are almost identical. The fine details of tooth position are governed by the final stages of mandibular movement into occlusion so that the teeth take up position with the retruded contact position and the intercuspal position almost the same. In a few people tooth malposition brought about by other factors results in the intercuspal position being very different from the position of initial contact. The usual mechanism for this will be discussed in the next section.

Mandibular movements

As with mandibular positions, movements of the mandible have an infinite variety. Although under voluntary control, they are usually the result of reflex activity initiated by sensory and proprioceptive receptors in the oral mucous membrane, periodontal tissues, temporo-mandibular joints and muscles of mastication and facial expression. The important movements to be considered here are those taking the mandible from the rest position, or from an adaptive postural position, to occlusion, as occurs during swallowing, and those which occur with the teeth in contact.

Mandibular closure

1   Normal closure

Normal closure of the mandible, which occurs in most people, takes the mandible from the rest position to the intercuspal position. It involves an upward and slightly forward movement of the mandible, and essentially a rotatory movement of the mandibular condyles in the articular fossae.

2   Closure from adaptive postural position

In closure from an adaptive postural position, the mandible usually moves directly from the postural position into the intercuspal position without any intermediate tooth contacts. The movement involved will depend on the position of the adaptive posture. In the most common forward posture the movement is upwards and backwards into occlusion.

3   Translocated closure

It has been mentioned previously that in a few people the intercuspal position is markedly different from the position of initial tooth contact. This is usually brought about by translocated, or deviated, closure from rest to occlusion. The common mechanism for this is that, during mandibular closure, lower teeth come into contact with one or more upper teeth before the intercuspal position is reached. Sensory and proprioceptive receptors in the periodontal tissues and in the masticatory muscles initiate a reflex mechanism which causes the mandible to deviate in its path of closure. The final intercuspal position is thus different from the position of initial contact.

A common example of translocated closure occurs when an upper lateral incisor erupts in palatal relation to the dental arch due to there being insufficient space within the arch. During closure of the jaws the lower incisor first comes into contact with the instanding upper incisor, and the mandible deviates forward or laterally. The teeth then meet in a position of maximum intercuspation which is different from the correct relationship, and, if uncorrected, the buccal teeth erupt into occlusion in the same position. Fig. 2.4 shows a gross example of translocated closure of the mandible.

Although translocated closure is brought about by premature contact of teeth in closure of the mandible, there appears to be a reflex protective mechanism which guides the mandible away from the premature contact before maximum force, or perhaps before any force, is exerted on the teeth in premature contact.

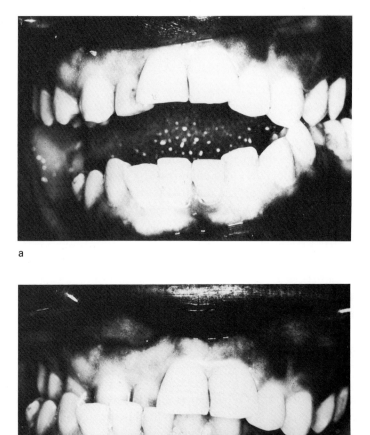

a

b

Fig. 2.4. Translocated closure of the mandible. (a) Initial contact of teeth on the left side of the jaws. (b) Movement of the mandible to the right to achieve maximum occlusion of the teeth.

Mandibular movements in occlusal contact (functional occlusion)

The full range of mandibular movement is much greater than that normally used for the purpose of mastication. Masticatory movements are essentially opening and closing movements of the jaw plus a combination of antero-posterior and lateral movements with the teeth in contact, the movements with occlusal contact being largely responsible for the actual breakdown of food by the teeth. Though under voluntary control, mastication is usually a reflex activity involving the muscles of the tongue, lips and cheeks as well as the muscles of mastication, the movements being initiated by sensory, proprioceptive and stretch receptors in the oral mucous membrane, periodontal tissues, muscles and temporo-mandibular joints.

In most dentitions, antero-posterior and lateral movements from the intercuspal position result in the loss of occlusal contact in part of the dental arch. In forward movement the lower incisors ride down the palatal slope of the upper incisors, bringing the posterior teeth out of contact (Fig. 2.5). In lateral movement the teeth on the side towards which the mandible moves remain in contact and the teeth on the opposite side become slightly separated. This loss of occlusal contact is less in dentitions which have undergone marked attrition so that the occlusal planes are relatively flat, but even in such dentitions some separation of the teeth usually occurs due to the slope of the anterior wall of the temporo-mandibular joint fossae and the downward movements of the mandibular condyle.

It is important for normal mastication that the teeth should be in the correct position for functional movement to occur without interference from misplaced teeth. If one or more teeth are in faulty positions, either through aberrant development or through restorative or orthodontic treatment, adverse tooth contacts may occur during masticatory movements. These contacts initiate reflex avoiding mechanisms of the mandible, which interfere with masticatory function and may give rise to periodontal or temporo-mandibular joint disease.

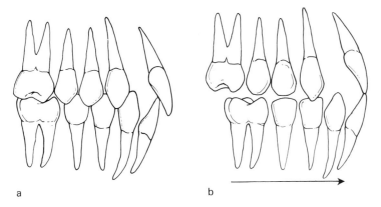

a   b

Fig. 2.5. Forward movement of the mandible. (a) Intercuspal position; (b) forward articulatory movement. The anterior teeth usually remain in contact but occlusal contact of the posterior teeth is lost.

Ideal occlusion

The concept that there is an ideal for each of the components of the occlusion of the teeth, from a knowledge of which variations, or mal-occlusions, can be measured, probably began with the work of Angle (1899), who, dealing strictly with static occlusion in the intercuspal position defined the ideal relationship of upper and lower first permanent molars in the sagittal plane. From this definition of the ideal, it was possible to define variations of the occlusion in the same plane, and Angle's classification of the occlusion, or modified versions of it, has been in widespread clinical use since it was devised (see p. 35).

Andrews (1972) outlined six keys to normal occlusion, derived from a study of 120 subjects whose ideal occlusions shared six features. The six features were related to:
1   Correct relationship of the first permanent molars in the sagittal plane.
2   Correct crown angulation of the incisor teeth in the transverse plane.
3   Correct crown inclination of the incisor teeth in the sagittal plane.
4   An absence of rotation of individual teeth.
5   Correct contacts of individual teeth within each dental arch, with no spacing or crowding.
6   A flat or only slightly curved occlusal plane.

Andrews postulated that if one or more of these features were incorrect, the occlusal relationships of the dentition could not be ideal.

Andrews' 'keys' again relate particularly to static occlusion, but define features not included in Angle's classification.

Some criteria for ideals of functional occlusion were outlined by Roth (1976). The following is a paraphase of Roth's concepts, which are directed towards the ensurance of the maximum masticatory efficiency consistent with the minimum traumatic loading on the teeth and supporting tissues and the muscular and skeletal masticatory apparatus.
1   In the position of maximum intercuspation (centric occlusion) the mandibular condyles should be in their most superior and most retruded position in the condylar fossae. This implies that the intercuspal position is the same as the retruded contact position.
2   On closure into centric occlusion, the stress on the posterior teeth should be directed along the long axes of the teeth.
3   The posterior teeth should contact equally and evenly, with no contact on the anterior teeth, in centric occlusion.
4   There should be minimal incisal overjet and overbite (see below), but sufficient to cause separation of the posterior teeth on any excursion of the mandible out of centric occlusion.

5   There should be minimal interference from the teeth to a full range of mandibular movement as limited by the temporo-mandibular joints.

Malocclusion of the teeth

Malocclusion can be said to exist in the following conditions.
1   When there is a need for the subject to take up an adaptive postural position of the mandible.
2   When there is translocated closure of the mandible from the rest position or from an adaptive postural position to the intercuspal position.
3   When the tooth positions are such that adverse reflex avoiding mechanisms are set up during masticatory function of the mandible.
4   When the teeth are causing damage to the oral soft tissues.
5   When there is crowding or irregularity of the teeth which may predispose to periodontal and dental disease.
6   When there is adverse personal appearance caused by tooth position.
7   When the position of the teeth interferes with normal speech.
These conditions provide the basis of the need for orthodontic treatment, which is aimed at altering the position and occlusion of the teeth.

The intercuspal position is commonly referred to as the occlusion of the teeth, and for the sake of convenience this convention will be observed in the following chapters. There are many varied conditions of occlusion, which may or may not constitute malocclusion, and the main variations can be classified.

Before discussing classification of the occlusion it is necessary to define some terms in common use.

Incisal overjet

The overjet is the horizontal distance between the upper and lower incisors in occlusion, measured at the tip of the upper incisor (Fig. 2.6). It is dependent on the inclination of the incisor teeth and the antero-posterior relationship of the dental arches. In most people there is a positive overjet, i.e. the upper incisor is in front of the lower incisor in occlusion, but the overjet may be reversed, or edge-to-edge (Fig. 2.6).

Incisal overbite

The overbite is the vertical distance between the tips of the upper and lower incisors in occlusion (Fig. 2.7). It is governed by the degree of

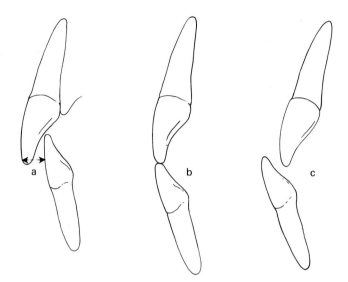

Fig. 2.6. Incisal overjet. (a) The ideal overjet relationship. (b) Edge to edge incisal position. (c) Reversed overjet.

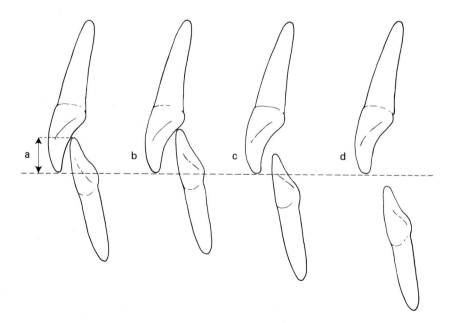

Fig. 2.7. Incisal overbite. (a) Ideal overbite relationship. (b) Excessive incisal overbite. (c) Incomplete overbite. (d) Anterior open bite.

vertical development of the anterior dento-alveolar segments. Ideally, the lower incisors contact the middle third of the palatal surface of the upper incisors in occlusion, but there may be excessive overbite, or there may be no incisal contact, in which case the overbite is described as *incomplete* when the lower incisors are above the level of the upper incisal edges, or *anterior open bite*, when the lower incisors are below the level of the upper incisal edges in occlusion (Fig. 2.7).

Transverse relationship

Overjet and overbite refer respectively to relationships in the sagittal and the vertical planes. In the transverse plane the posterior teeth also have ideal relationships which are subject to variation. In the ideal relationship the upper teeth should overlap the lower teeth on both sides (see Fig. 3.1). A common variation is the development of a *buccal crossbite* on which the lower posterior teeth are buccally placed in relation to the upper teeth (see Fig. 3.22a). Less common is the development of a *lingual crossbite*, with the lower teeth lingually placed in relation to the upper teeth (see Fig. 3.22b). Both types of crossbite vary in degree, and may be unilateral or bilateral.

Classification of the occlusion of the teeth

The following classification is based on that of Edward Angle (1899), though differing in some important respects. It is a classification of the antero-posterior relationship of the upper and lower dental arches, and does not take into account lateral and vertical relationships, crowding and local malposition of teeth.

Class 1

The accepted ideal relationship. It is an antero-posterior relationship such that, with the teeth in their correct positions in the dental arch, the tip of the upper canine tooth is on the same vertical plane as the distal edge of the lower canine tooth. The upper premolar teeth interdigitate in a similar manner with the lower premolar teeth, and the antero-buccal cusp of the upper first permanent molar occludes in the mesial buccal groove of the lower first permanent molar (Fig. 2.8). If the incisor teeth are in their correct inclination, the incisal overjet is about 3 mm.

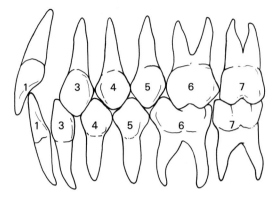

Fig. 2.8. Class 1 occlusion. The accepted ideal occlusal relationship.

Class 2

In the Class 2 relationship, the lower dental arch is more posterior to the upper dental arch than in Class 1 relationship. It is therefore sometimes called *'post-normal relationship'*. Two types of Class 2 relationship are commonly seen, and the class is therefore subdivided.

Class 2 Division 1

The dental arches are in Class 2 relationship, the upper central incisors are proclined and the incisal overjet is increased (Fig. 2.9). The upper lateral incisors may also be proclined.

Class 2 Division 2

The dental arches are in Class 2 relationship, the upper central incisors are retroclined and there is an increased incisal overbite (Fig. 2.9). The upper lateral incisors may be proclined or retroclined.

It is not always possible to place a Class 2 occlusal relationship into one of these divisions, in which case the occlusion may be designated *'indefinite Class 2'*.

Class 3

In the Class 3 relationship the lower dental arch is more anterior to the upper dental arch than in the Class 1 relationship. It is therefore

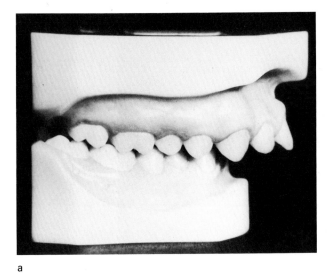

a

b

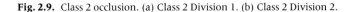

Fig. 2.9. Class 2 occlusion. (a) Class 2 Division 1. (b) Class 2 Division 2.

sometimes called *'prenormal relationship'* (Fig. 2.10). Two main types of Class 3 relationship are seen. In the first, usually called *'true Class 3'* the lower jaw moves from the rest position into Class 3 occlusion with a normal closure. In the second, the incisors are so positioned that mandibular closure causes the lower incisors to contact the upper

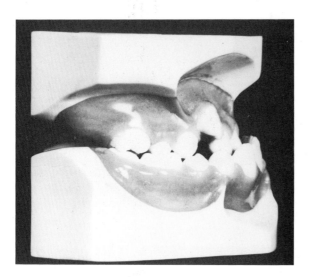

Fig. 2.10. Class 3 occlusion.

incisors before centric occlusion is reached. The mandible therefore moves forward in a translocated closure into the intercuspal position. This type of relationship is usually called *'postural'* or *'displacement' Class 3* (Fig. 2.11).

In any type of occlusal relationship local tooth malposition may be superimposed on the basic relationship of the dental arches. Thus the detail of the intercuspation of the teeth may not correspond with the overall classification of the dental arch relationship. If many teeth are malpositioned it may be difficult or impossible to classify the occlusion. Furthermore, asymmetries may cause the relationship on one side of the jaws to be different from that on the other. In these circumstances it is necessary to describe the occlusion in words, rather than in the verbal shorthand of a classification.

It seems likely that the proportions of occlusions falling into the various categories described above differs in different populations. In a study of the dental occlusion in a population of Shropshire school children in the age range 11 to 12 years, Foster and Day (1974) found the following approximate proportions.

Class 1	44%
Class 2 Division 1	27%
Class 2 Division 2	18%
Class 2 (indefinite)	7%

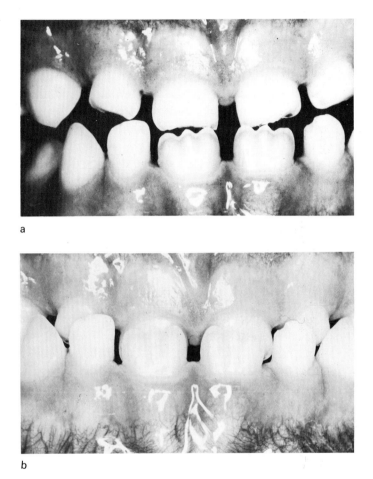

a

b

Fig. 2.11. Postural Class 3 occlusion. (a) In closure from the rest position the incisor teeth meet edge-to-edge, with the buccal teeth apart. (b) The mandible is postured forward into a Class 3 occlusion.

Class 3 (true)	3%
Class 3 (postural)	0.3%

It can be seen from this that although Class 1 occlusal relationship is the ideal, it was not necessarily the normal, comprising less than half the population.

The quantification of malocclusion

It will be seen that the foregoing classifications of malocclusion are entirely descriptive, and do not contain any indication of the degree of discrepancy. In clinical diagnosis and treatment planning as well as in epidemiological studies it is usually necessary to measure or estimate the degree of occlusal variation. Incisal overjet and overbite can be measured directly, with added description of 'complete' or 'incomplete' for overbite. However, since the incisor teeth differ in length between individuals, the degree of overbite is often estimated in terms of the degree of coverage of the lower incisor by the upper incisor in the vertical plane in occlusion. Similarly, since the width of the posterior teeth differs between individuals, it is convenient to describe discrepancy in relationship between upper and lower posterior teeth in the sagittal plane in terms of *units*, a unit being the width of the first upper premolar tooth of the individual concerned.

Buccal and lingual crossbites can be measured, but are more usually described in words. The degree of crowding or spacing of the dental arches can also be measured by measuring the difference between the total sum of the widths of the individual teeth and the size of the arch which is available to contain them. For clinical treatment purposes, however, it is more customary to divide the arches into four quadrants and to quantify crowding of the arches in terms of *units* of one first premolar width, for each quadrant. Other occlusal aberrations, such as rotation and malposition of individual teeth, are usually described in words and quantified where possible.

Malocclusion and the masticatory apparatus

It is tempting to believe that any departure from the ideals of static and functional occlusion is likely to lead to disorders of the other components of the masticatory apparatus, particularly the temporo-mandibular joint and the masticatory muscles. This does not seem likely to be the case as far as natural occlusion is concerned. Many studies have been carried out on patients with temporo-mandibular joint and muscle dysfunction. Most investigators agree that the problem has a multifactorial aetiology, with malocclusion being one possible factor, but that no single factor is both necessary and sufficient to cause the problem. Conversely, studies of malocclusion have largely failed to find a definitive correlation between the type or severity of a malocclusion and temporo-mandibular dysfunction (Helm *et al.* 1984; McLaughlin 1988). It may, however, be possible to produce occlusal dysfunction by means of orthodontic treatment, and there is a growing awareness that, in addition to attempting to achieve the ideals of static occlusion, orthodontic treatment should have good functional occlusion as one of its objectives. Howat and Spary (personal communication 1989) have outlined the functional aspects of the occlusion which should be present at the completion of orthodontic treatment. These are:

1 Centric occlusion should be the same as centric relation to avoid postural deviations.

2 There should be maximum possible tooth contact in centric occlusion, in order to spread periodontal stress.

3 Incisal guidance should separate the buccal teeth on mandibular protrusion.

4 There should be group function on protrusion, i.e. the lower six anterior teeth should all be in contact with upper incisors.

5 In lateral movement, there should be no occlusal contacts on the balancing side.

6 On the working side in lateral movement there should be canine contact only.

Summary

Static occlusion

The static contact of upper and lower teeth.

Functional occlusion

The dynamic movement of the lower jaw with teeth in contact.

Mandibular positions

1 Non-occlusal

(a) Rest position—muscles relaxed; maintained by stretch reflex.
(b) Adaptive postural positions—to achieve oral seal or oral respiration.

2 Occlusal

(a) Retruded contact position—centric relation—the occlusal position with the mandibular condyles in the most posterior position.
(b) Intercuspal position—centric occlusion—the position of maximum intercuspation of the teeth.

Mandibular movements

Though under voluntary control, they are largely reflex movements.

1 Mandibular closure

(a) Normal closure—movement from rest position to intercuspal position—usually upward and forward.
(b) Closure from adaptive postural positions—usually upward and backward.
(c) Translocated closure—deviation caused by premature tooth contacts.

2 Functional movement

Only part of the dentition usually remains in occlusion.
(a) Forward—incisors remain in contact.
(b) Lateral—contact remains on the side towards which movement is directed.

Reflex avoiding mechanisms may be caused by misplaced teeth, leading to adverse tooth contacts.

Ideal occlusion

Accepted ideals exist for both static and functional occlusions.

Malocclusion

The presence of adaptive postural positions, translocated closures, reflex avoiding mechanisms, crowding, irregularity of the teeth, dental trauma to soft tissue and adverse personal appearance or interference with normal speech caused by tooth position.

Occlusal classification

A classification of antero-posterior relationship of the dental arches.
CLASS 1. Ideal antero-posterior dental arch relationship.
CLASS 2. Lower dental arch in posterior relation to upper arch.
 Division 1. Upper central incisors proclined, increased incisal overjet.
 Division 2. Upper central incisors retroclined, increased incisal overbite.

CLASS 3. Lower dental arch in anterior relation to upper arch.

Postural Class 3. Translocated forward closure of the mandible into Class 3 relationship.

In any of these types of occlusion there may be lateral or vertical discrepancies in dental arch relation, or crowding or irregularity of the teeth.

Measurement of occlusal discrepancy

Direct measurement of overjet and overbite. Measurement of posterior sagittal relationship and crowding in units. Descriptive quantification of other irregularities.

Orthodontic treatment and occlusion

At the end of treatment, the functional as well as the static occlusion should be correct.

References

Andrews, L. F. (1972) The six keys to normal occlusion. *Am J Orthod,* **62**, 296–309.

Angle, E. H. (1899) Classification of malocclusion. *Dent Cosmos,* **41**, 248–264.

Foster, T. D. & Day, A. J. W. (1974) A survey of malocclusion and the need for orthodontic treatment in a Shropshire school population. *Br J Orthod,* **1**, 73–78.

Helm, S., Kreiborg, S. & Solow, B. (1984) Malocclusion at adolescence related to self-reported tooth loss and functional disorders in adulthood. *Am J Orthod,* **85**, 393–400.

McLaughlin, R. P. (1988) Malocclusion and the temporo-mandibular joints. *Angle Orthod,* **58**, 185–191.

Roth, R. H. (1976) The maintenance system and occlusal dynamics. *Dent Clin North Am,* **20**, 761–788.

3

The development of the occlusion of the teeth

Orthodontic treatment deals with alteration of the occlusion and position of the teeth. That this is necessary stems from the fact that there is a wide range of normal variation possible in the dental occlusion. In the next chapter the sources of occlusal variation will be outlined. In this chapter the development of the occlusion will be described, both from the point of view of ideal development and of the more common variations which occur. As with growth of the jaws, it should be important, in planning orthodontic treatment, to have a knowledge of the developmental changes which have occurred in the occlusion, whether the situation is improving or deteriorating, whether prognosis for change with growth is favourable or unfavourable and what changes might ensue following interference with the occlusion at any particular stage of development. Up to now, the extent of variation in development has made it difficult to apply such considerations to orthodontic practice, though a good deal of investigation is in progress.

Ideal development of the occlusion of the primary dentition

The primary dentition begins to erupt at the age of about 6 months, and is normally completely in occlusion by about 3 years of age. Details of mean age of eruption and the range of variation have been reported by Van der Linden (1983), by Hägg and Taranger (1985) for Swedish children and by Sato and Ogiwara (1971) for Japanese children. There appear to be no significant differences between the sexes for the age of primary tooth eruption.

The first teeth to erupt and to form occlusal contacts are the incisors, which ideally take up occlusal positions as illustrated in Fig. 3.1. The ideal position of the primary incisors has been described as being more vertical than the permanent incisors, with a deeper incisal overbite. The lower incisors in this condition will contact the cingulum area of the upper incisors in centric occlusion. Spaces are present between the primary incisor teeth.

Following eruption of the incisors, the first primary molars erupt into occlusion. These teeth take up occlusal contacts so that the lower molar is slightly forward in relation to the upper molar (Fig. 3.1).

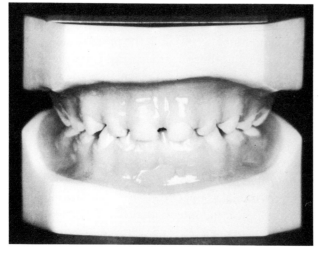

a

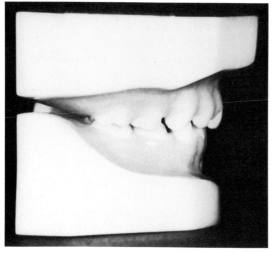

b

Fig. 3.1. The accepted ideals of occlusion of the primary dentition. The anterior teeth are spaced, there is a positive incisal overbite and overjet, the anthropoid spaces are present and the distal surfaces of the second molar teeth are in the same vertical plane.

The canine teeth are next to reach occlusion. In the ideal situation, a space exists mesial to the upper canine and distal to the lower canine, into which the opposing canine tooth interdigitates (Fig. 3.1). Such spaces are a normal feature of the permanent dentition in the higher apes, and in the human primary dentition are usually referred to as the anthropoid spaces.

The last teeth to erupt into occlusion in the primary dentition are the second molars. These teeth erupt slightly spaced from the first molars, but the space quickly closes by forward movement of the second molars, which take up a position so that the distal surfaces of the upper and lower second molars are in the same vertical plane in occlusion (Fig. 3.1).

Thus certain features of the 'ideal' occlusion of the primary dentition when fully erupted can be described viz:

1   Spacing of incisor teeth.
2   Anthropoid spaces mesial to upper canine and distal to lower canine, into which the opposing canine interdigitates.
3   Vertical position of incisor teeth, with lower incisor touching the cingulum of upper incisor.
4   The distal surfaces of the upper and lower second primary molars in the same vertical plane.

Variation in the occlusion of the primary dentition

Although it is possible to describe ideals for the position of the primary teeth, it is unusual to find those ideals all existing together in any one individual. A study of the occlusion of the teeth between $2\frac{1}{2}$ and 3 years of age (Foster & Hamilton 1969) revealed that out of 100 children studied, not one matched up to all four ideals previously listed. The main variations were as follows:

1   Only 33% of the children had spacing between all the incisor teeth. In 3%, no spaces existed in the incisor teeth and a further 3% had crowding of the incisor teeth. The remainder had spaces between some of the incisors, in various positions (Fig. 3.2).
2   The anthropoid space was absent in the upper arch in 13% and in the lower arch in 22% of the children. This feature appears to be the most constant of the 'ideals' in the primary dentition.
3   The incisal overbite matched up to the ideal in only 19% of the children. There was a reduced overbite in 37%, an anterior open bite in 24% and an excessive overbite, with the lower incisors occluding on the palate, in 20% (Fig. 3.3).
4   Only 55% of the children had the distal surfaces of the upper and lower primary molars on the same vertical plane. In 26% the lower molars were further back than the upper molars, and in 4% the lower

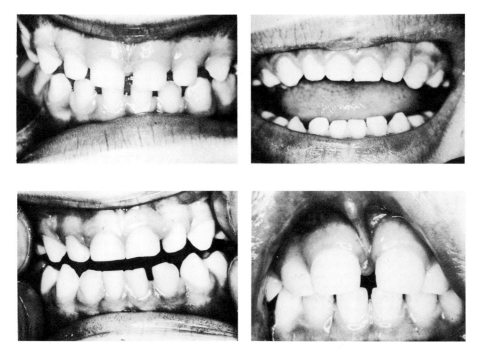

Fig. 3.2. Variation in spacing of the primary incisors at $2\frac{1}{2}$ years of age.

molars were further forward than the upper molars. In the remainder, the relationship differed between the two sides.

5 Excessive incisal overjet was present in 72% of the children (Fig. 3.4). In some cases this resulted from the lower dental arch being positioned further back than the upper arch. In others, the variation arose from the very common habit of thumb sucking, which tended to procline the upper incisors and retrocline the lower incisors.

Changes in the occlusion and position of the primary dentition after eruption

Once the teeth have erupted into occlusal contact, their position in relation to each other cannot be regarded as static. Changes occur in tooth position and occlusion during growth of the head, and as with the initial positions, these changes exhibit variation. Certain concepts which were formerly held regarding changes in the primary dentition are probably incorrect. Changes in the primary dentition can be categorized as follows:

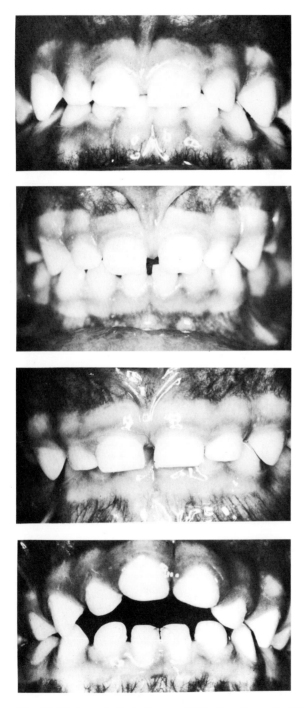

Fig. 3.3. Variation in the incisal overbite in the primary dentition at $2\frac{1}{2}$ years of age.

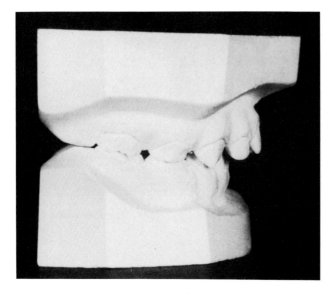

Fig. 3.4. Excessive incisal overjet at $2\frac{1}{2}$ years of age. In this case the relationship of the primary molar teeth is correct.

Changes in spacing condition

There is little change in the spacing or crowding condition of the primary dentition apart from the early closure of the space between the first and second molars, although in some children there appears to be a late spacing of the incisors immediately prior to these teeth being exfoliated (Fig. 3.5). Apparent spacing of the incisors may also occur as a result of occlusal attrition, the wider incisal part of the teeth being worn away to leave apparently larger spaces between the narrower remaining parts.

Changes in incisor relationship

Studies of changes in incisor relationship during the period of the primary dentition have been carried out by Foster *et al.* (1972) among others. There is general agreement that the mean changes include a reduction in incisal overjet and overbite. Reduction in overjet has usually been thought to be associated with forward growth of the mandible during this period. Reduction in overbite has been associated with the attrition of the teeth which occurs to a marked degree in the primary dentition, and to differential growth of the alveolar processes of the jaws.

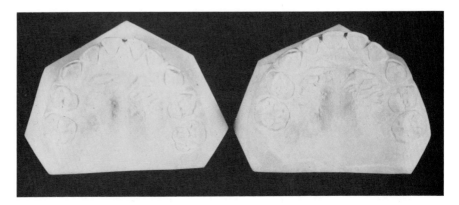

Fig. 3.5. Closure of molar spaces in the primary dentition. (*Left*) On eruption at about $2\frac{1}{2}$ years, the second molars are often spaced from the first molars. (*Right*) One year later, the molar spaces have usually closed, while the other spaces in the dentition remain unchanged.

However, although there is a mean reduction in overjet and overbite, there is considerable individual variation in these changes. Foster *et al.* (1972) studying changes in individual children between $2\frac{1}{2}$ and $5\frac{1}{2}$ years of age, found that while 72% of the children showed a decrease in overjet, 25% showed an increase and 3% showed no change in overjet. Changes in incisal overbite were even more variable, with 52% showing a decrease, 44% an increase and 4% no change. These variations may be related to thumb and finger sucking habits, which are so common in young children (Fig. 3.6).

As previously mentioned, the primary teeth undergo marked

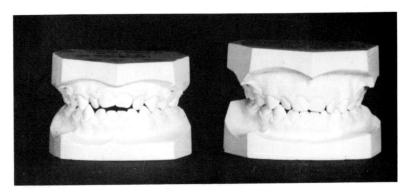

Fig. 3.6. Spontaneous closure of anterior open bite in the primary dentition, probably as a result of stopping the thumb sucking habit. (*Left*) $2\frac{1}{2}$ years. (*Right*) $3\frac{1}{2}$ years of age.

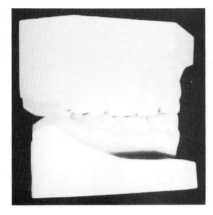

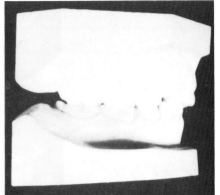

a

b

Fig. 3.7. Forward posture of the mandible in the primary dentition at $5\frac{1}{2}$ years of age. (a) Attrition of the teeth enables the mandible to be moved forward with all the teeth in occlusion. The correct occlusion is shown in (b). The models (c) show the occlusion in the mixed dentition.

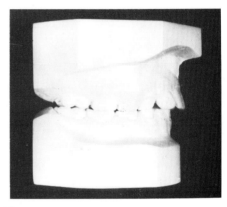

c

attrition of the occlusal and incisal surfaces between the time of eruption and exfoliation. As a result of this, by the age of about $5\frac{1}{2}$ years, the occlusal table of the primary dental arches is relatively smooth, with freedom from cuspal interdigitation. This often allows the mandible to be postured forward so that the incisor teeth are in an edge-to-edge occlusion, while the buccal teeth are still in complete occlusal contact. Such a situation has led to the misconception that an edge-to-edge incisor relationship is a 'normal' feature of the occlusion at this stage. Foster *et al.* (1972) found that only about 5% of children studied has an edge-to-edge incisor occlusion at the age of $5\frac{1}{2}$ years, and it seems likely that such an occlusion is a postured position in most children, the true occlusal relation being with the mandible in a more retruded position, and with a positive incisal overjet (Fig. 3.7).

Changes in antero-posterior dental arch relationship

It has commonly been thought that the usual change in antero-posterior relationship of the dental arches in the primary dentition is a forward translation of the lower arch in relation to the upper. However, studies of individual changes (Foster *et al.* 1972) have suggested that, as with the incisor relationship, there is no consistent pattern of change in the antero-posterior dental arch relationship, and indeed the most common tendency is for no change to occur at all between $2\frac{1}{2}$ and $5\frac{1}{2}$ years of age. The antero-posterior relationship of the upper and lower primary canine teeth showed no change in 50% of the children studied, and changes in the remainder varied between a forward movement and a backward movement of the mandibular canine in relation to the maxillary canine. Similar results were found on studying the changes in the relationship between the distal surfaces of the upper and lower second primary molars.

Changes in dental arch dimensions

It is generally agreed that the dimensions of the dental arches change very little during the period of the established primary dentition. Foster *et al.* (1972) found a slight increase in the mean dimensions of the dental arches between $2\frac{1}{2}$ and $5\frac{1}{2}$ years of age, but there was individual variation, with some children showing no increase and a small number showing decrease in dimensions.

Development of the occlusion of the permanent dentition

From the age of about 6 years onwards the primary dentition is replaced by the permanent dentition. The primary incisors, canines and molars are replaced by the permanent incisors, canines and premolars, and the permanent molars erupt as additional teeth.

There is some difference in size between the primary teeth and the permanent teeth which directly replace them. The permanent incisors and canines are usually larger than the corresponding primary teeth, and the premolars are usually smaller than the corresponding primary molars. Studies reported by Van der Linden (1983), have shown that the overall difference in size between the two dentitions is not large, amounting on average to about 3 mm in the upper teeth and less than 1 mm in the lower teeth. There is, however, not a strong correlation between the sizes of the primary dentition and the successional permanent dentition, particularly for the lower incisors and there is considerable individual variation. In addition there is the need to accommodate three extra teeth, the permanent molars, in each quadrant of the jaws, and the tendency for the teeth to move forward to make space in conditions of potential crowding.

The extra size of the permanent successional dentition and the need to accommodate the permanent molars probably account for the fact that crowding is much more common in the permanent dentition than in the primary dentition.

In ideal development, the extra size of the permanent dentition is accommodated through two factors.

1   The primary dentition is spaced

If the primary teeth erupt with incisor spacing there is a better chance that the permanent teeth will not be crowded than if the primary teeth erupt without incisor spacing. Foster and Grundy (1986) have shown that with no spacing of the primary teeth there is a 75% chance of crowding of the successional permanent teeth. However, individual variation may result in crowding of permanent teeth even following a spaced primary dentition particularly if the permanent teeth are excessively large in relation to the primary teeth (Fig. 3.8) (Sampson & Richards 1985).

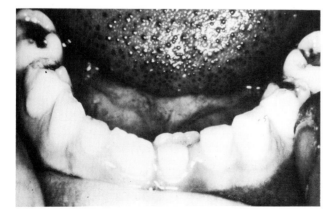

Fig. 3.8. Excessively large permanent teeth may be crowded even though the primary teeth are spaced. In this case, the permanent central incisors will occupy all the available extra space and the permanent lateral incisors will be crowded.

2 The dental arch increases in size

Studies have shown that increase in size of the dental arch is mainly concomitant with tooth eruption. Such increase in size obviously takes place with increase in jaw growth in all dimensions but particularly in lateral and antero-posterior dimension.

Ideal development of the occlusion of the permanent dentition, and some common variations

The development of the occlusion of the permanent dentition can be regarded as having three stages.
1 Eruption of first permanent molars and incisors.
2 Eruption of canines, premolars and second molars.
3 Eruption of third molars.

The tooth which does not fit well into this scheme is the lower canine tooth, which, erupting at about 9 years of age, comes between the first and second stage. The eruption times for the permanent dentition and the usual variation range have been reported by Van der Linden (1983) and by Hägg and Taranger (1985) for Swedish children. In general, eruption times are somewhat earlier in girls than in boys, but they are likely to vary slightly between different populations.

Stage 1

The first stage in development is concerned with the replacement of the primary incisor teeth and the addition of the four first permanent molars to the dentition. This usually occurs in the age range 6–8 years. The permanent incisors erupt slightly more proclined than the primary incisors, and therefore have less incisal overbite when they reach occlusal contact. This proclination also plays a part in increasing the size of the dental arch.

Eruption of the first permanent molars occurs early in the development of the permanent occlusion, usually at the age of about 6 years. These teeth initially meet in occlusion in such a position that the distal surface of the upper molar is on the same vertical plane as the distal surface of the lower molar. Later, with the loss of the second primary molars, the lower first permanent molar will move forward more than the upper first permanent molar, so that the distal surface of the lower first permanent molars will be slightly anterior to that of the upper molar, and the antero-buccal cusp of the upper molar will occlude in the

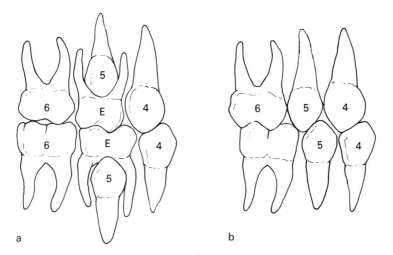

a   b

Fig. 3.9. (a) In ideal development, the first permanent molars initially meet in a Class 2 relationship. (b) Following loss of the second primary molars, the lower first permanent molar moves forward into the ideal Class 1 relationship.

mesial buccal groove on the lower molar (Fig. 3.9). The reason for this differential forward movement is that the upper and lower premolars are much the same width, whereas the lower second primary molar is wider in mesio-distal dimension than the upper second primary molar.

Variations from ideal development in Stage 1

The ideal development described above is all too rare. Furthermore, several investigators have pointed out the variability and unpredictability of the changes from primary to permanent dentition occlusion (Foster & Grundy 1986; Bishara *et al.* 1988; Leighton & Feasby 1988). The following variations are commonly seen.

1   Variation in spacing and crowding conditions

Crowding of the teeth is a common feature of most mixed populations, and is often first manifested at the stage of eruption of the permanent incisors. Crowding of the permanent incisor teeth involves the lateral incisors more frequently than the central incisors. The central incisors usually erupt first, and occupy space which should be available for the lateral incisors. The lateral incisors then have to erupt in a crowded position, commonly rotated, instanding or protruded (Fig. 3.10). Sometimes, of course, the central incisors are also crowded (Fig. 3.11).

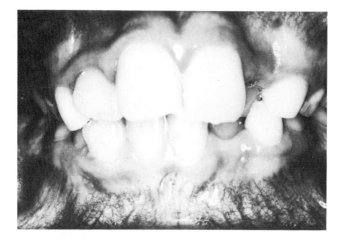

Fig. 3.10. Crowding in the anterior region affecting the permanent lateral incisors, the central incisors having erupted first and taken up most of the available space.

Crowding of the dental arches occasionally affects first permanent molar eruption, usually by causing impaction of the first permanent molar against the distal surface of the second primary molar (Fig. 3.12).

2   Variation in antero-posterior relationship

The ideal antero-posterior relationship of the incisor teeth and the first permanent molars is not by any means always achieved during

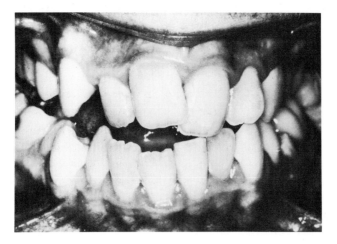

Fig. 3.11. Crowding affecting permanent central incisors.

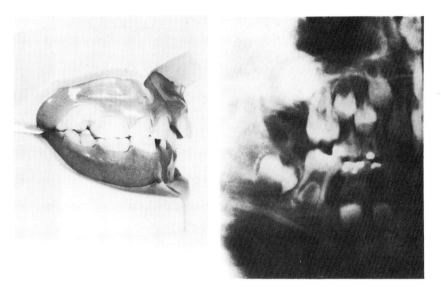

Fig. 3.12. Crowding affecting first permanent molar eruption in the upper arch.

development of the dentition. The reasons for this will be discussed in the next chapter. At this stage it can be said that commonly, the lower incisors achieve their initial occlusal position further back or further forward than the ideal, in relation to the upper incisors (Figs. 2.9, 2.10). This may be associated with variation in the inclination of these teeth, which are sometimes retroclined, sometimes proclined compared with the ideal inclination. Similarly, the initial occlusal relationship of the first permanent molars varies in the antero-posterior dimension (Figs. 2.9, 2.10).

3 *Variation in vertical relationship*

While the first permanent molars usually reach occlusal contact, there is a wide range of variation in the vertical relationship of the incisor teeth. Development in the vertical plane may cease before the incisors reach occlusal contact, and this is usually due to the intervention of the thumb or tongue (Fig. 3.13). On the other hand, there may be excessive vertical development of the anterior dento-alveolar segments so that there is an excessive overbite with the teeth in occlusion. This is usually associated with variation in inclination of the teeth, particularly retroclination of upper and/or lower incisors, or variation in the antero-posterior relationship so that the teeth do not reach normal occlusal

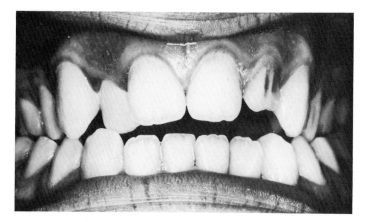

Fig. 3.13. Asymmetrical anterior open bite, the result of finger sucking preventing the full vertical development of the anterior dento-alveolar segments.

contacts and therefore the dento-alveolar structures continue to develop (see Fig. 2.7b).

4 Variation in lateral relationship

Variation in the lateral position of the upper incisors in relation to the mid-sagittal plane is sometimes seen. In this condition the permanent central incisors are each tilted distally, so that there is a space between the crowns of the teeth (Fig. 3.14). The apices of the teeth may be close together, and this may be due to there being insufficient space for the teeth to be accommodated on the basal bone of the jaws. This condition may also be due to pressure from the erupting lateral incisors and canines, and sometimes resolves when these teeth erupt into the dental arch.

The first permanent molars may also develop into aberrant lateral relationships, with the lower molars occluding too far laterally or medially in relation to the upper molars.

5 Localized variation in tooth position

Apart from the general variations in development in Stage 1 mentioned above, a wide range of variation is possible in individual tooth position. Such variations have a variety of causes, which will be discussed later, including the presence of supernumerary teeth, retained primary incisors due to infection, early trauma causing malposition of the

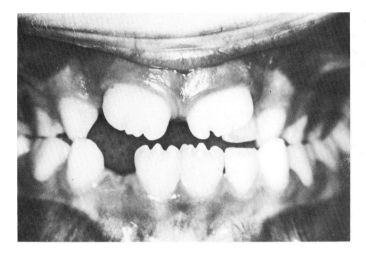

Fig. 3.14. Distal tilting of erupting permanent upper central incisors.

developing permanent incisor and aberrant developmental position of teeth (Fig. 3.15).

Stage 1 is usually completed by the end of the ninth year, and soon after this the permanent lower canine teeth erupt, replacing the corresponding primary teeth. the main variation in development at this

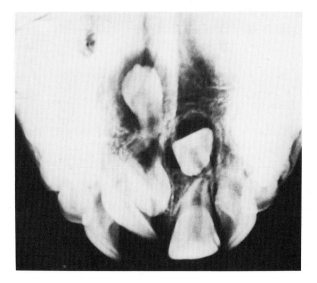

Fig. 3.15. Variation in position of developing teeth. Supernumerary teeth and aberrant position of the permanent upper canine are seen in this radiograph.

stage is caused by crowding, when there is insufficient space for the permanent canine teeth to be accommodated in the dental arch. In this condition, the canine teeth usually erupt in buccal relationship to the arch, and may be inclined mesially or distally (Fig. 3.16).

Stage 2

The second stage in the development of the occlusion of the permanent dentition is concerned with the replacement of the primary molars and upper canine teeth by the premolars and permanent upper canines, and

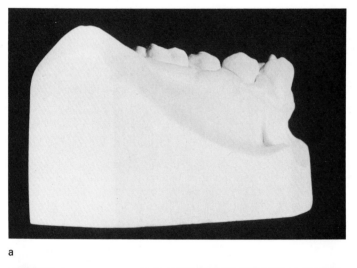

a

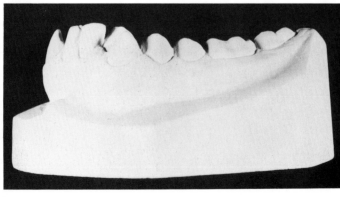

b

Fig. 3.16. Lower permanent canine teeth malpositioned due to lack of space in the arch, showing (a) mesial, and (b) distal inclination of canines.

the addition of the second molar teeth. This usually takes place in the age range 10–13 years.

The first premolars are usually the first teeth to erupt in this stage, and meet in occlusion so that the distal slope of the occlusal surface of the lower premolar occludes with the mesial slope of the occlusal surface of the upper premolar. Thus the tip of the cusp of the upper premolar will be in the same vertical plane as the distal surface of the lower premolar (see Fig. 2.8). The second premolars then erupt into a similar relationship, and at about the same time the upper canine tooth erupts into occlusion so that the tip of its cusp is on the same vertical plane as the distal surface of the lower canine. Thus each upper buccal tooth, in occlusion, is a half tooth-width more posterior than the corresponding lower tooth. This is the Class 1 occlusal relationship previously described (see Fig. 2.8).

Finally the second molars erupt into an occlusion similar to that of the first molars. The upper second molar develops high in the alveolar process, immediately below the floor of the maxillary antrum. Initially it usually has a slight distal tilt, and it has a longer eruptive path than the lower second molar. The lower second molar usually develops in an upright position, or with a slight mesial tilt (Fig. 3.17). Thus the upper

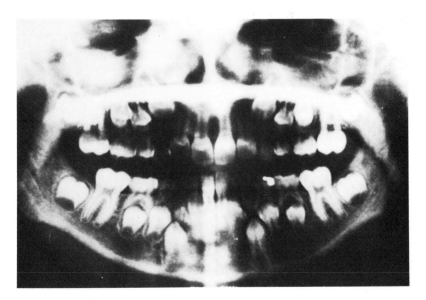

Fig. 3.17. Developmental position of the second permanent molars. The upper molars are usually slightly tilted distally and have a greater tendency to move forward during eruption than the lower molars.

second molar has a greater tendency to move forward during eruption than the lower second molar, which has a relatively short and straight eruptive path.

Variations from ideal development in Stage 2

The more common variations in development in Stage 2 are as follows:

1   Variation due to crowding

Crowding of the dental arches frequently provides a source for variation. As with the incisor teeth, it particularly affects the last teeth to erupt, in this stage either the second premolar or the upper canine tooth. If the second premolar has not enough space to erupt in its correct position in the dental arch it usually erupts in palatal or lingual relation to the arch (Fig. 3.18). Similarly, the upper canine tooth may erupt in an aberrant position due to crowding, in this case usually in buccal relation to the arch (Fig. 3.19). Sometimes either the second premolar or the upper canine tooth will be impacted against other teeth and will fail to erupt, due to there being insufficient space (Fig. 3.20).

2   Variation in antero-posterior relationship

The antero-posterior relationship of the occlusion of the premolars and canines is subject to variation, though the range of variation is less than that of the incisors. This is because the incisors have greater facility for proclination or retroclination than the buccal teeth. However, the lower buccal teeth may be further back or further forward than their ideal occlusal relationship with the upper teeth, i.e. they may be in Class 2 or Class 3 relationship (see Figs. 2.9, 2.10).

3   Variation in vertical relationship

The only variation in vertical relationship which is possible in the buccal teeth is that they fail to meet when other teeth are in occlusion. This is not common, and when present is usually due to intervention of the tongue, which prevents the full development of the dento-alveolar structures (Fig. 3.21).

4   Variation in lateral relationship

The lateral relationship of the premolars and canines in occlusion can vary. Aberrant lateral positions of these teeth due to crowding has

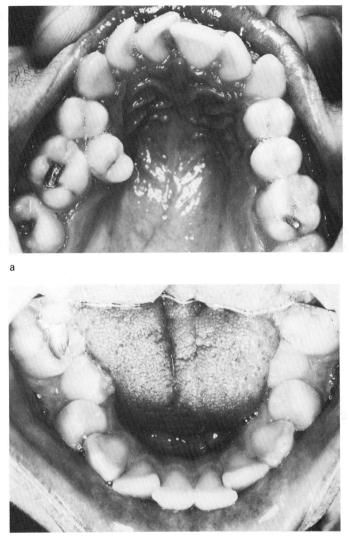

a

b

Fig. 3.18. The second premolar usually erupts in a lingual direction if there is insufficient space in the arch.

already been mentioned and is perhaps the most usual variation in lateral relationship. Variation due to other causes, notably differences in size between upper and lower jaws, will be discussed later. The upper buccal teeth may be in medial relation to the lower teeth, giving the so-called crossbite (Fig. 3.22), or less commonly, the lower teeth may be in medial relation to the upper teeth (Fig. 3.22b).

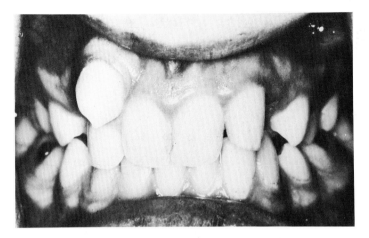

Fig. 3.19. Crowding of the arch often causes the upper canine to erupt on the buccal aspect of the arch.

5 Localized variation in tooth position

There is a smaller range of localized variation in tooth position in the buccal teeth than in the incisors. The one possible exception to this general statement is the upper permanent canine tooth, which exhibits an aberrant developmental position more frequently than any other

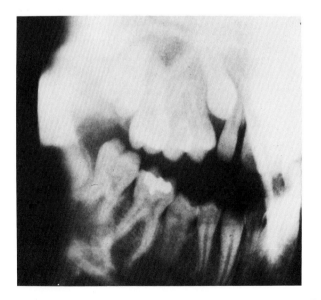

Fig. 3.20. Radiograph showing impacted upper canine with insufficient space to erupt into the arch.

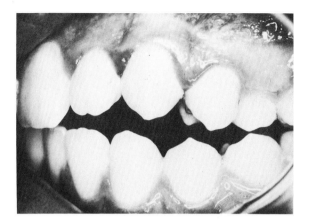

Fig. 3.21. Lateral open bite due to intervention of the tongue between the developing upper and lower dento-alveolar structures.

tooth except the lower third molar. It has been said that this is because the upper canine tooth has a longer path of eruption than most other teeth, but this is doubtful. Both upper and lower canine teeth have a longer path of eruption than other teeth in their respective jaws (Fig. 3.23), but the upper tooth is much more commonly malpositioned than the lower. Furthermore, the upper canine tooth can sometimes be seen to be in an aberrant position at an early stage in its development, and although this is sometimes spontaneously corrected during eruption it is sometimes progressive. It is more usual to find an aberrant upper canine tooth developing and erupting on the palatal side of the dental arch than on the buccal side, unless the tooth is forced to erupt on the buccal side of the arch because of lack of space in the arch.

The variations in the eruptive path of the permanent upper canine are not completely understood at present. The tooth should cause resorption of the root of the primary canine if it is to erupt into correct position, but although it may appear not to be doing this, the tooth may nevertheless finally move to its correct position in relation to the other teeth (Fig. 3.24).

Stage 3

The eruption of the third molars in early adult life completes the development of the occlusion of the permanent dentition. The usual age range for third molar eruption is 18–25 years, although they can erupt slightly earlier or much later than this.

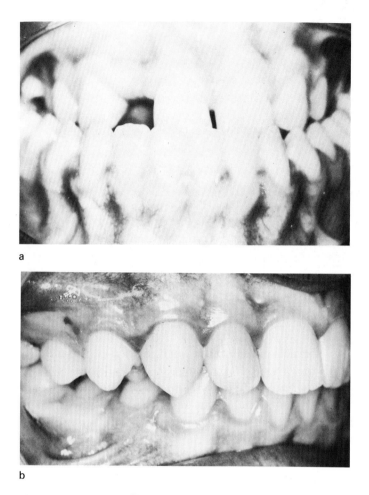

a

b

Fig. 3.22. (a) Buccal crossbite. (b) Lingual occlusion of the lower premolars.

The third molars develop in much the same position as the second molars, with the upper third molar developing high, under the postero-inferior corner of the maxillary antrum, and usually with a slight distal inclination. The lower third molar has a shorter path of eruption than the upper, and is initially positioned more vertically, or with a slight mesial inclination. The two teeth erupt into occlusion in a similar relationship to that of the first and second molars.

Variations from ideal development in Stage 3

Variation in antero-posterior relationship and lateral relationship can occur in Stage 3 as in the previous stages, but the main variations in

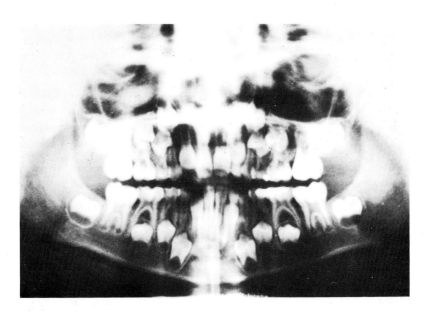

Fig. 3.23. Developmental position of permanent canine teeth. The upper and lower canines develop higher and lower respectively than any other teeth.

third molar development are those due to crowding and to the developmental position of the teeth, with these two causes often being combined in one individual.

1 Variation due to crowding

The third molar is the last tooth to erupt, and frequently has not enough space to erupt into its correct occlusal position. In the lower jaw this results in the tooth becoming impacted vertically between the second molar and the anterior ascending ramus of the mandible, and failing to erupt completely. In the upper jaw, the third molar usually erupts, even in crowded conditions, but may erupt on the posterior or lateral aspect of the upper alveolar process and will not be in occlusion with the lower third molar.

2 Variation due to developmental position

The lower third molar, perhaps more than any other tooth, has a tendency to develop in an aberrant position. More commonly it has a mesial inclination, sometimes to the extent of developing horizontally, but a variety of other positions are possible. The mesial inclination

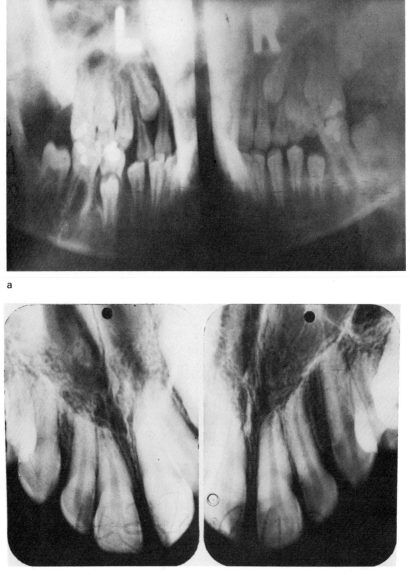

a

b

Fig. 3.24. Development of the permanent upper canine tooth. Although the permanent canine often appears to be mesial to the primary canine at an early stage in development (a); it can nevertheless erupt into a normal position (b). Radiographs of the same patient at 9 years and 13 years of age.

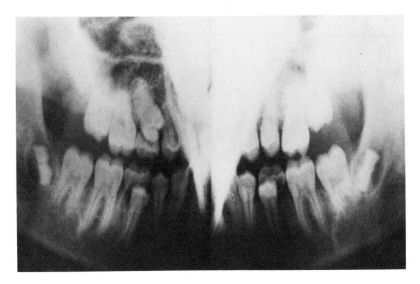

Fig. 3.25. Mesial inclination of the developing lower third molars.

usually causes the tooth to be impacted against the second molar, and prevents its eruption into occlusion (Fig. 3.25).

Mesial migration of teeth

The development of the occlusion of the teeth is accompanied by movement of the dentition in the vertical, lateral and antero-posterior planes. As the jaws increase in size, the teeth are carried downward, forward and laterally in the maxilla, and upward, forward and laterally in the mandible, by means of alveolar growth. The forward movement of the dentition during development has been called *physiological mesial migration* of the teeth. It has been suggested that such movement takes place throughout life, but there is probably some confusion between forward movement during development and the tendency for teeth to move forward in certain circumstances after eruption (see Chapter 6). Forward movement of teeth during growth has been illustrated by Brash (1924), who showed, by madder-feeding experiments on pigs, that alveolar bone growth is accompanied by mesial movement of the teeth, bone being resorbed from the sockets in front of the teeth and new bone being added to the sockets behind the teeth. Although there is much greater forward growth of the jaws in the pig than in man, concomitant with the development of the snout, it seems likely that similar forward movement of the dentition occurs in man during growth, though to a lesser degree.

It should be noted that this normal forward movement of the whole dentition will not result in the closure of spaces between the teeth. Closure of spaces is associated with a different type of mesial movement of teeth, which occurs after eruption and which seems to be particularly associated with the dentition being of excessive size in relation to the size of the dental arch. This latter type of mesial movement can occur after growth has ceased and in some circumstances can occur throughout life, given that there is opportunity for the teeth to move. Such opportunity is usually made in modern times by the loss of teeth, leaving spaces into which other teeth can move. In more primitive communities the space was frequently made by interproximal attrition of the teeth through the coarse texture of the diet. Begg (1954), from measurements of Australian aboriginal teeth, has estimated that as much as 14.7 mm might be lost from the total mesio-distal length of the dentition of the lower jaw by interproximal attrition by the time the third molars erupt. This loss of tooth substance is compensated by the forward movement of teeth so that interproximal contacts are maintained. Lysell (1958) has found, from a study of mediaeval skulls, that such attrition and forward movement of individual teeth may be progressive throughout life. In a large jaw, however, with spaces between the teeth, this type of mesial movement of individual teeth obviously does not occur, otherwise the spaces would close.

Thus, two types of mesial movement of teeth occur.
1 Mesial movement of the dentition as a whole, as part of dento-alveolar forward development during growth. This type of movement can be regarded as the physiological mesial migration.
2 Mesial movement of individual teeth into spaces created either by loss of teeth or by interproximal attrition. This type of mesial movement is particularly associated with a large dentition in relation to size of the dental arch (see Chapter 6).

Changes during the development of the permanent dentition

It is important to realize that the permanent dentition does not erupt into a static unchanging environment. During the 6 or 7 years over which most of the permanent occlusion develops, growth is continuing and maturation of function is occurring. The jaws are enlarging, particularly in the vertical dimension, and the jaws and dentition are undergoing translative growth in a downward and forward direction in relation to the base of the skull. This growth may exhibit a differential between the posterior and the anterior components of the jaws, resulting in rotation of the jaws and contained dentition (Björk & Skeiller 1983). Changes in activity of the orofacial muscles result in different forces being applied to the teeth. The adoption or cessation of habits, particularly the cessation of thumb sucking, may alter the form of the dental arches. The eruption of teeth may cause increase in crowding and irregularity of the teeth, and the eruption of teeth into aberrant positions may cause premature occlusal contacts to develop, with subsequent translocated closure of the mandible and altered occlusion. Differential jaw growth may change the occlusal relationship, as sometimes happens when a puberal mandibular growth spurt increases the degree of Class 3 relationship or decreases the degree of Class 2 relationship.

This potential for change makes it desirable to have a knowledge of any changes which have occurred and are occurring during the development of a child's occlusion, so that any orthodontic treatment can be planned in the light of such knowledge.

Summary

Occlusion of the primary dentition

This develops between 6 months and 36 months of age.

Ideal positions

1 Incisors spaced.
2 Anthropoid spaces—mesial to upper canine, distal to lower canine.
3 Incisors vertical, lower incisors occluding on cingulum of upper incisors.
4 Distal surfaces of upper and lower second molars in the same vertical plane.

Variation

1 Spacing inconsistent.
2 Anthropoid spaces not always present, though the most persistent feature.

3 Overbite variable; may be excessive, incomplete or anterior open bite.

4 Overjet variable; frequently excessive.

5 Terminal plane of molars variable.

Changes in primary occlusion

Usually marked attrition of teeth.

Main positional changes

1 No change in spacing condition except closure of molar spaces.

2 Slight reduction in overbite and overjet, though considerable individual variation.

3 No consistent pattern of change in antero-posterior dental arch relationship.

4 Little change in dental arch dimensions.

Occlusion of permanent dentition. This develops from 6 years onwards. Successional permanent teeth slightly larger in total than primary teeth. In addition, permanent molars have to be accommodated. Extra space made by:

1 Spaced position of primary teeth.

2 Increase in dental arch size concomitant with tooth eruption.

Stages of ideal development

There are three stages of ideal development:

Stage 1

Eruption of incisors and first molars, 6–8 years. Incisors more proclined than primary incisors. First molars initially occlude with distal surfaces in same vertical plane. Lower moves forward more than upper when primary second molar exfoliated.

Stage 2

Eruption of canines, premolars and second molars, 10–14 years.

Stage 3

Eruption of third molars, 18–25 years.

Variations

1 Spacing and crowding condition. Crowding more common, usually affecting lateral incisors, canines, second premolars and third molars.
2 Antero-posterior relationship. May develop Class 2 or Class 3 relationship. Variation in incisor inclinations.
3 Vertical relationship. Variation in incisal overbite and relationship of buccal teeth.
4 Lateral relationship. Development of crossbite.
5 Individual tooth position. Upper canines and lower third molars particularly liable to aberrant developmental position.

There are two types of mesial movement of teeth.
1 Mesial movement of the dentition during development.
2 Mesial movement of individual teeth to close spaces made by tooth loss or attrition.

Changes during development caused by growth, maturation of muscle function, alteration in habits or eruption of teeth, may cause changes in occlusal relationships.

References

Begg, P. R. (1954) Stone-age man's dentition. *Am J Orthod*, **40**, 298–312.

Bishara, S. E., Hoppens, B. J., Jakobsen, J. R. & Kohout, F. J. (1988) Changes in the molar relationship between the deciduous and the permanent dentitions: a longitudinal study. *Am J Orthod*, **93**, 19–28.

Björk, A. & Skeiller, V. (1983) Normal and abnormal growth of the mandible: a synthesis of longitudinal cephalometric implant studies over a period of 25 years. *Eur J Orthod*, **5**, 1–46.

Brash, J. C. (1924) The growth of the jaws and palate. In *The Growth of the Jaws in Health and Disease*. London, Dental Board of the United Kingdom.

Foster, T. D., Grundy, M. C. & Lavelle, C. L. B. (1972) Changes in occlusion in the primary dentition between $2\frac{1}{2}$ and $5\frac{1}{2}$ years of age. *Eur Orthod Soc Trans*, 75–84.

Foster, T. D. & Grundy, M. C. (1986) Occlusal changes from primary to permanent dentitions. *Br J Orthod*, **13**, 187–193.

Foster, T. D. & Hamilton, M. C. (1969) Occlusion in the primary dentition. *Br Dent J*, **126**, 76–79.

Hägg, U. & Taranger, J. (1985) Dental development, dental age and tooth count. *Angle*

Orthod, **55**, 93–107.

Leighton, B. C. & Feasby, W. H. (1988) Factors affecting development of molar occlusion: a longitudinal study. *Br J Orthod,* **15**, 99–103.

Lysell, L. (1958) Qualitative and quantitative determination of attrition and the ensuing tooth migration. *Acta Odontol Scand,* **16**, 267–292.

Sampson, W. J. & Richards, L. C. (1985) Prediction of mandibular incisor and canine crowding changes in the mixed dentition. *Am J Orthod,* **88**, 47–63.

Sato, S. & Ogiwara, Y. (1971) Eruption order of deciduous teeth. *Bull Tokyo Dent Coll,* **12**, 45–76.

Van der Linden, F. P. G. M. (1983) In *Development of the Dentition.* Chicago, Quintessence Publishing Co.

4

Skeletal factors affecting occlusal development

It can be seen from the previous chapters that the final form of the occlusion and position of the teeth exhibits a wide range of variation. The main factors responsible for producing this variation can be divided into two groups, the first group containing major factors which have a general effect on the occlusion and which play a part in the development of every occlusion, and the second group containing more localized factors, which do not appear in everyone, but which nevertheless may be the main factor in producing a malocclusion in an individual. The factors can be grouped as follows:

General factors affecting occlusal development

1 *Skeletal factors.* The size, shape and relative positions of the upper and lower jaws.
2 *Muscle factors.* The form and function of the muscles which surround the teeth, i.e. the muscles of the lips, cheeks and tongue.
3 *Dental factors.* The size of the dentition in relation to the size of the jaws.

Local factors affecting occlusal development

1 Aberrant developmental position of teeth.
2 The presence of supernumerary teeth.
3 Hypodontia—the congenital absence of certain teeth.
4 The effects of certain habit activities.
5 Localized soft tissue anomalies—the labial frenum.

The general factors will always be present, producing ideal occlusion or some occlusal variation, and usually the three major factors are interrelated. Thus the muscles are attached to the jaws, and variation in jaw position may produce variation in muscle action. Similarly variation in muscle activity may alter the relevance of variation in the size of the dentition. The local factors may be present in isolation or in combination, and may be superimposed on the adverse effect of one or more of the general factors, adding further complications to the occlusion of the

teeth.

It is proposed to discuss each of these factors separately, and to outline its effect on the dental occlusion.

Skeletal factors affecting occlusal development

Any pathological condition affecting growth of the jaws is likely to have a marked effect on the occlusion of the teeth. Inherited and acquired congenital malformation, trauma or infection during the growing years can all affect jaw growth (Fig. 4.1). However, this book is concerned not with pathological conditions, which are relatively uncommon, but with normal variation, which is frequent and wide-ranging. Only normal variation will therefore be considered.

The teeth are appendages of the jaws and are supported by the alveolar bone, which in turn is based on the basal bone of the jaws (Fig. 4.2). The division of the jaw bones into basal and alveolar components is artificial, as both obviously belong to the same bone. Nevertheless, it is convenient to accept this division, as the two parts behave differently in

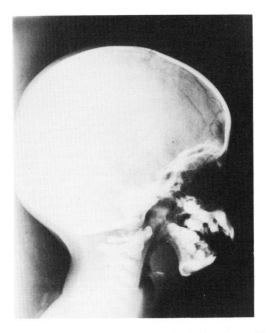

Fig. 4.1. Lateral skull radiograph of a child with mandibulo-facial dysostosis, an inherited condition in which growth of the facial bones is defective. The severe effect on the occlusion can be seen.

development and function, and perhaps the concept of the jaws having various functional components is desirable. Indeed, the basal component may be further subdivided on a functional basis but this may not be relevant to the subject of occlusal variation.

As the teeth are set in the jaws, the relationship of the jaws to each other will have a large influence on the relationship of the dental arches.

Jaw relationship can be considered under three headings:

1   Jaws in relation to the cranial base.
2   Jaws in relation to each other.
3   Alveolar bone in relation to basal bone.

Jaws in relation to cranial base

The jaws are part of the total structure of the head, and it is possible for each jaw to vary in its positional relationship to other structures of the head. Such variation can exist in all three planes, sagittal, lateral and vertical, but is usually greatest in the sagittal and vertical planes. It is usual in orthodontic diagnosis to relate the jaw positions to the anterior cranial base, and each jaw can vary independently in its relationship to the cranial base.

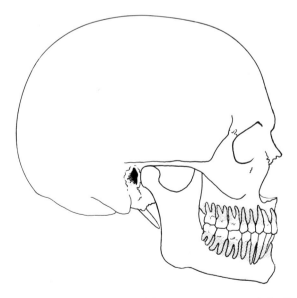

Fig. 4.2. The components of the jaws can conveniently be divided into alveolar bone, (shaded) which invests the teeth, and basal bone, which forms the main structure of the jaws.

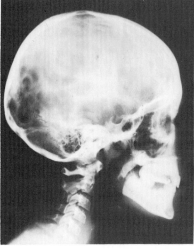

a

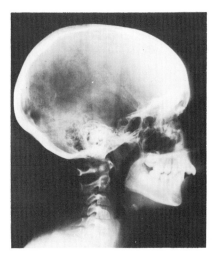

b

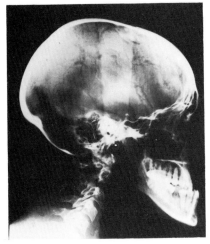

c

Fig. 4.3. The skeletal relationship of the jaws. (a) skeletal Class 1; (b) skeletal Class 2; (c) skeletal Class 3.

Jaws in relation to each other

The relationship of the jaws to each other can also vary in all three planes of space, and variation in any plane can affect the occlusion of the teeth.

The *antero-posterior* positional relationship of the basal parts of the upper and lower jaws to each other, with the teeth in occlusion, is known as the *skeletal relationship*. This is sometimes called the dental

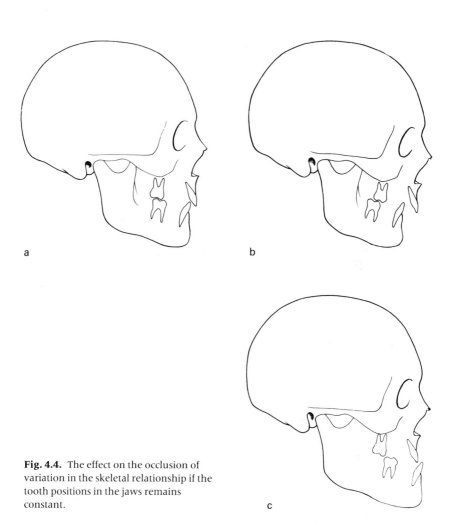

a

b

Fig. 4.4. The effect on the occlusion of variation in the skeletal relationship if the tooth positions in the jaws remains constant.

c

base relationship, or the skeletal pattern. A classification of the skeletal relationship is in common use, namely:

1   Skeletal Class 1—in which the jaws are in their ideal antero-posterior relationship in occlusion.

2   Skeletal Class 2—in which the lower jaw in occlusion is positioned further back in relation to the upper jaw than in skeletal Class 1.

3   Skeletal Class 3—in which the lower jaw in occlusion is positioned further forward than in skeletal Class 1.

Examples of Class 1, 2 and 3 are shown in Fig. 4.3. There is, of course, a range of severity of skeletal Class 2 and Class 3.

Fig. 4.4 shows the effect of variation of the skeletal relationship on the occlusion of the teeth if the tooth position in the jaw remains constant.

Variation in the skeletal relationship can be brought about by:

1   Variation in size of the jaws.

2   Variation in position of the jaws in relation to the cranial base.

Thus if one jaw is excessively small or large in relation to the other in antero-posterior dimension the development of skeletal Class 2 or Class 3 relationship may result (Fig. 4.5). Furthermore if one jaw is set further back or further forward than the other in relation to the cranial base, again a skeletal Class 2 or Class 3 relationship may result.

The relative sizes of the jaws in lateral dimension also has an effect on the occlusion of the teeth. Ideally the jaws match in size, so that the occlusion of the buccal teeth in transverse relation is correct. Occasionally one jaw is wider than the other to such an extent that the occlusion of the teeth is affected, giving a buccal crossbite (see Fig. 3.22a) if the lower jaw is wider, or lingual occlusion of the lower teeth (see Fig. 3.22b) if the upper jaw is wider. Buccal crossbite may be unilateral or bilateral, and will be described in more detail in a later chapter.

The vertical relationship of the upper and lower jaws also affects the occlusion. The effect is most clearly seen with variation in the shape of the lower jaw at the gonial angle. The mandible with a high gonial angle

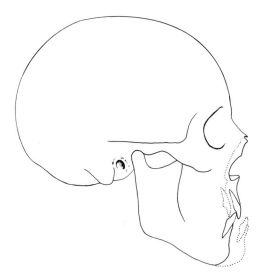

Fig. 4.5. Variation in the size of either jaw can affect the skeletal relationship. Skeletal Class 3 resulting from a small upper jaw or from a large lower jaw.

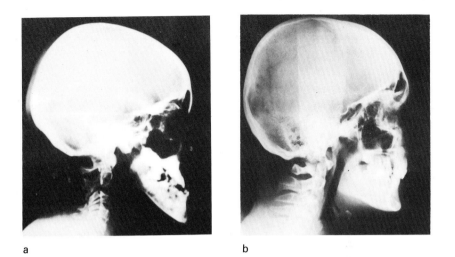

a   b

Fig. 4.6. The effect of variation of the gonial angle on facial height. At the extremes of the range of normal variation a high gonial angle (a) tends to produce a large facial height and a low gonial angle (b) a small facial height.

tends to produce a longer vertical dimension of the face, and in severe cases an anterior open bite. Conversely, the mandible with a low gonial angle tends to produce a shorter vertical dimension of the face (Fig. 4.6).

Alveolar bone in relation to basal bone

The term 'skeletal relationship' refers to the basal bone of the jaws. Although the alveolar bone is supported by the basal bone, the relationship between the upper and lower alveolar bones is not necessarily the same as that between the upper and lower basal bones. The alveolar bone supports the teeth, and will therefore match tooth position rather than basal bone position. Nevertheless, the basal bone provides the base, and the alveolar bone relationships, and hence the tooth relationships, can only differ from the basal relationships within a limited range. This is a very important factor in orthodontic treatment.

The reason for the possibility of difference between alveolar and basal relationships is that tooth position is not governed entirely by jaw position. Other factors, to be discussed later, may cause the teeth, during eruption, to be tilted away from their correct inclinations. Alveolar bone grows to support the tilted teeth, and therefore may be slightly different in position from the basal bone (Fig. 4.7). However, the teeth cannot be moved completely away from the basal bone during eruption. Therefore

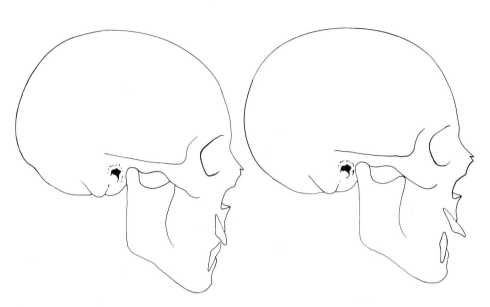

Fig. 4.7. Tooth and alveolar bone position may to a limited extent be independent of skeletal relationship. In this illustration the skeletal relationship is the same in each case, but different inclinations of the teeth within the jaws has produced different occlusal relationships.

it is the basal bone relationships which are most important in occlusal development.

The skeletal relationship in orthodontic treatment

The skeletal relationship is not only important in the part it plays in occlusal development. It also plays a major part in orthodontic treatment. It seems likely that orthodontic treatment which is confined to tooth movement has little effect on the size, shape or relative positions of the basal parts of the jaws. Its only direct effect is on tooth position and on alveolar bone position and form. Therefore, as the teeth must be positioned on the basal bones, the skeletal relationship must limit the amount of tooth movement which can be achieved. In particular, the skeletal relationship limits the amount of antero-posterior movement of the incisor teeth, and it may not be possible to correct incisor positions in Class 2 or Class 3 occlusal relationship if they are based on severe Class 2 or Class 3 skeletal discrepancies.

In practical terms, it is relatively easy to alter the inclination of the incisor teeth, producing little or no change in the position of the apices of the teeth. Treatment techniques are available which can produce

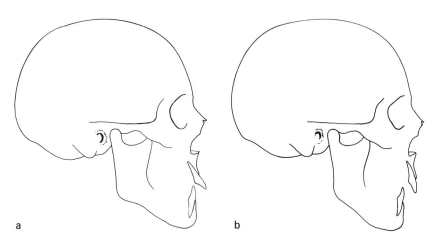

a   b

Fig. 4.8. Although the skeletal relationship in (a) and (b) are different, the incisal overjets are similar, due to variation in incisal inclination.

apical movement, and this can to some extent, overcome skeletal discrepancies. Even these techniques however, are limited in their scope, and the severe skeletal discrepancy remains a limiting factor to orthodontic treatment. Fig 4.8 shows two similar occlusions, each with the same degree of increased incisal overjet, but based on different skeletal patterns. It would be more difficult to reduce the incisal overjet in the occlusion based on the Class 2 skeletal relationships (Fig. 4.8b), where the teeth are in the correct inclination, than in the occlusion based on the Class 1 skeletal relationship (Fig. 4.8a), where the increased overjet has been produced by proclination of the upper incisor teeth.

Assessment of the skeletal relationship

As the skeletal relationship plays a major part in determining the occlusal relationship, and as it is also a major limiting factor in orthodontic treatment, it is necessary to be able to assess it accurately on the individual patient.

The skeletal relationship may be assessed by clinical or by radiographic methods.

Clinical assessment

Some idea of the skeletal relationship can be gained simply by observation of the subject in profile. The gross discrepancies may be

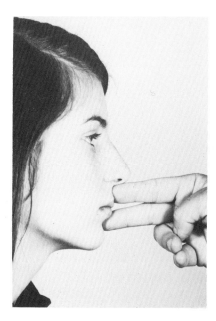

Fig. 4.9. The assessment of skeletal relationship by palpation.

assessed in this way, but the less marked discrepancies may be masked by tooth position or by the thickness or posture of the lips. A more accurate impression can be obtained by palpation of the anterior surface of the basal part of the jaws, with the teeth in occlusion (Fig. 4.9). Although the thickness of the lips may interfere with the assessment, this method can give a reasonable impression of the skeletal relationship.

A clinical method of assessment in common use is based on a study of the inclination of the incisor teeth and the degree of incisal overjet. It presumes that if the inclinations of the upper and lower incisor teeth are correct, with an ideal skeletal relationship (Class 1) there will be an ideal incisal overjet of about 2–3 mm. This assumes that, as the incisor teeth erupt into the mouth, they may be tilted forward or backward by the various pressures to which they are subjected, such as pressures from lips and tongue, but their apices remain in a fairly stable position on the basal bone. If this assumption is correct, then the degree of incisal overjet will depend on: (a) the degree of incisal inclination; and (b) the antero-posterior relationship of the apical bases, i.e. the skeletal relationship.

This method of assessing the skeletal relationship is therefore:
1 Assess the inclination of the upper and lower incisors.
2 Assess the degree of incisal overjet which is present.

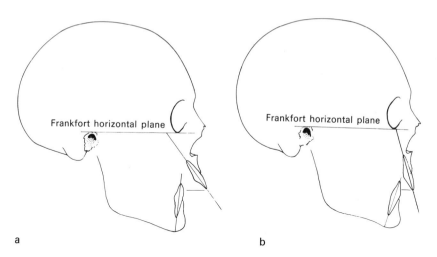

a   b

Fig. 4.10. The method of residual overjet for clinical assessment of the skeletal relationship. (a) The clinical appearance of the patient, with proclined upper and retroclined lower incisors, and a grossly excessive overjet. (b) The estimated correct inclination of the incisors, with the apical positions unchanged. The overjet is now only slightly excessive, indicating a slight degree of skeletal Class 2 relationship.

3   If the teeth are not in their correct inclinations, assess the degree of incisal overjet which would be present if the teeth were realigned to their correct inclinations, without moving the apices of the teeth.

The *'residual overjet'* gives an indication of the skeletal relationship, an excessive residual overjet indicating a skeletal Class 2 and a reduced or reversed residual overjet indicating a skeletal Class 3. The degree of residual overjet also indicates the degree of skeletal discrepancy.

Fig. 4.10 illustrates this method of assessment.

The method of residual overjet may give a reasonable assessment of the skeletal relationship in many cases. Its accuracy, however, is open to question, since it depends on the assumption that the incisor teeth do not move to any great extent in relation to the basal bone, apart from changing in inclination. Furthermore, it is sometimes difficult to assess the true incisor inclination from a clinical view of the crowns of the teeth.

Radiographic assessment

While clinical assessment, if carefully carried out, can give a reasonably accurate picture of the skeletal relationship, radiographic assessment is without doubt more accurate. It is based on the method of standardized cephalometric radiography pioneered by Broadbent (1931). The purpose of this radiographic technique is to produce standardized radiographs of the head, and the equipment consists of a cephalostat, which holds the head in a predetermined position, an X-ray tube and a film. These three components are maintained in a fixed relationship to each other, so that any angulation and magnification is standardized and any films produced by one piece of equipment are comparable with each other. The cephalostat contains two ear-rods which fit into the external auditory meati of the subject, and the X-ray tube and film are aligned so that, when filming a lateral view of the head, the central beam of the X-rays passes through the two ear pieces and is at right angles to the film. The source of the rays is usually set at a distance of 150 cm or more from the subject in order to minimize the magnification (Figs. 4.11, 4.12). The cephalostat can be rotated in the horizontal plane to obtain any view of the head, but for assessment of the skeletal relationship the lateral view is used. Standardized radiographs of this sort are used in longitudinal studies of growth of the head, for comparisons of size and form between individuals or groups and for individual assessment of form, usually in orthodontic treatment planning or in assessing the results of treatment procedures.

In the cephalometric assessment, certain carefully defined points are located on the radiograph, and linear and angular measurements are made from these points. The expression of these measurements in various ways produces analyses of skeletal size and form. Traditionally

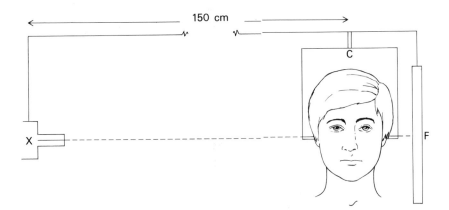

Fig. 4.11. Diagrammatic representation of the cephalometric radiographic technique. The central ray passes through the ear-rods of the cephalostat, and is perpendicular to the film. The distance from the X-ray source to the cephalostat is at least 150 cm in order to minimize magnification. X = X-ray source, C = cephalostat, F = film.

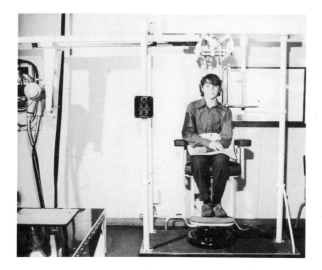

Fig. 4.12. Patient in position for cephalometric lateral skull radiography, showing the position of the X-ray tube (*left*), cephalostat and film.

the point location and measurements have been performed simply by tracing outlines on the skull radiograph and measuring by hand, but systems are now available and in wide use for computer analysis of skeletal form after the manual plotting of co-ordinates on the radiograph. More recently, methods of automatic scanning of radiographs are being developed, to avoid the need for manual point location, which is the source of most of the errors in cephalometric methods.

There are many systems of cephalometric analysis, which utilize various points and outlines on the radiograph. The following is a list of some of the more commonly used reference points, and the radiographic assessments of the skeletal relationship to be described use some of these points and lines.

Some cephalometric points and lines located on the lateral skull radiograph (Fig. 4.13)

Cephalometric points

- *Porion.* The highest point on the margin of the external auditory meatus.
- *Orbitale.* The lowest point on the infra-orbital margin.
- *Nasion.* The junction of nasal and frontal bones in the mid-line.
- *Sella.* The centre of the shadow of sella turcica.

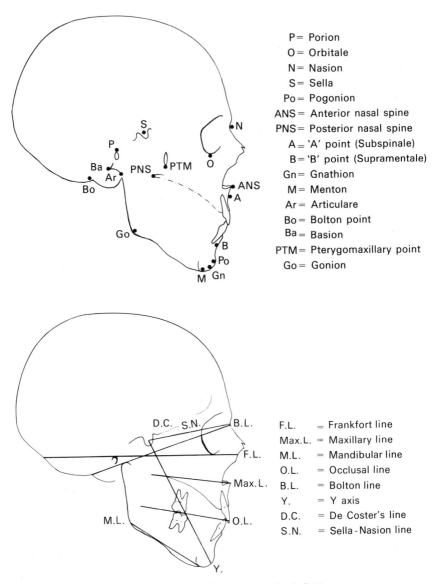

Fig. 4.13. Some cephalometric points and lines. See text for definition.

- *Pogonion.* The most anterior point on the bony chin.
- *Anterior nasal spine (ANS).* The most anterior projection of the premaxilla in the mid-line below the nasal cavity.
- *Posterior nasal spine (PNS).* The most posterior projection of the hard palate in the mid-line.

- *Point A (subspinale).* The most posterior point of the concavity on the anterior surface of the premaxilla in the mid-line, below the anterior nasal spine.
- *Point B (supramentale).* The most posterior point of the concavity on the anterior surface of the mandible in the mid-line, above the pogonion.
- *Gnathion.* The most inferior and anterior point on the bony chin, where the bisector of the angle made by the vertical and horizontal tangents to the chin meets the mandibular outline.
- *Menton.* The most inferior point on the lower border of the mandible where the shadow of the lower border of the mandible meets the shadow of the cross-section of the mandibular symphysis.
- *Gonion.* The most inferior and posterior point at the angle of the mandible, where the bisector of the angle between tangents to the posterior and inferior borders of the mandible meets the mandibular outline.
- *Articulare.* The point of intersection of the outlines of the posterior border of the mandible and the inferior border of the temporal bone.
- *Bolton point.* The highest point in the concavity of the fossa behind the occipital condyle.
- *Basion.* The lowest point on the anterior margin of the foramen magnum in the mid-line.
- *Pterygomaxillary point.* The lowest point of the outline of the pterygo-maxillary fissure.

It will be appreciated that some of these points are in the mid-sagittal plane, and are therefore single points, while others, such as gonion and articulare, are bilateral points. On a true lateral radiograph the bilateral points should be superimposed, and should appear as a single point, but owing to facial asymmetries this is not always the case. If any bilateral points appear separately on the radiograph, it is conventional to accept a point halfway between the two as being the correct position.

The significance of certain points should also be appreciated. The lines nasion–sella and sella–basion broadly represent the slope of the centre of the anterior and middle cranial bases respectively. Point A and point B represent the anterior surfaces of the tooth-supporting dental bases of the maxilla and mandible. The pterygomaxillary point at the posterior surface of the maxillary antrum, represents the posterior end of the tooth bearing area of the maxilla. Other points are joined to form cephalometric lines, which are used for measurement and alignment of the head in growth and other studies.

Cephalometric lines

It has been conventional for many years to refer to the various reference lines constructed by joining points on lateral skull radiographs as cephalometric planes. However, since a plane has two dimensions while a line drawn on a radiograph has only one dimension, it is more accurate to refer to cephalometric lines. The following is a descriptive list of the more commonly used reference lines. There are many different systems of cephalometric analysis, and other reference lines are sometimes used.

Frankfort line. The line joining the orbitale and the porion on the left side. This is accepted by convention as the horizontal line of the head, and is commonly used for orientation of the head in clinical and radiographic assessments.

Maxillary line. The line joining the anterior nasal spine and the posterior nasal spine. This line is sometimes used instead of the Frankfort line in radiographic assessment, particularly as the Frankfort line is sometimes difficult to locate accurately on a radiograph. However, the maxillary line does not bear any fixed relationship to the Frankfort line, and the two lines are not usually parallel (Foster *et al.* 1981). The maxillary line cannot, of course, be assessed clinically.

Mandibular line. The line joining gonion and menton. It represents the line of the lower border of the mandible, and can roughly be assessed clinically.

Sella–nasion line. The line joining the centre of the sella turcica and the nasion. It is used to represent the anterior cranial base, to which the position of the jaws and teeth are often related in cephalometric analysis.

Facial line. The line joining nasion and pogonion. The angular relationship between the facial line and the Frankfort line is used as a measurement of mandibular prognathism.

Occlusal line. The line from the mid-point between the tips of the upper and lower incisors to the anterior contact between the upper and lower first molars in occlusion.

Bolton line. The line joining the Bolton point and the nasion.

Y axis. The line from sella to gnathion.

De Coster's line. The outline of the internal surface of the anterior cranial base from the anterior lip of the sella turcica to the endocranial surface of the frontal bone (De Coster 1952).

Three further reference lines are sometimes used, particularly in treatment planning, to assess the aesthetic qualities of the facial profile and tooth positions.

The *A–pogonian line* (Williams 1969) is a line joining A point and the pogonion. It is claimed that in ideal skeletal and occlusal form the incisal tips of the lower central incisors should lie on or near to this line. It is a useful guide in treatment planning, but it must be remembered that this line does not necessarily represent a position of stability for the lower incisors, particularly if the skeletal relationship in the sagittal plane is not ideal.

The *aesthetic line* (Ricketts 1957) is a line joining the most anterior points of the tip of the nose and the chin. It is claimed that, for good aesthetic profile qualities, the anterior border of both upper and lower lips should lie on or close to this line.

The *Holdaway line* (Holdaway 1983) is a line joining the anterior borders of the upper lip and the chin. Again, it is claimed that for good aesthetic profile qualities the anterior border of the lower lip should lie on or close to this line.

It will be appreciated that the last two lines mentioned above have soft tissue landmarks and relate to lip position. They are therefore subject to soft tissue variation, such as lip muscle thickness and tone, and although they will be modified by variation in the skeletal relationship, variation in tooth position will have a relatively smaller effect. Furthermore, they are related to aesthetic qualities, and beauty is in the eye of the beholder.

Superimposition of lateral skull radiographs

In the assessment of growth or treatment changes in dento-facial form, it is often necessary to superimpose successive radiographs of one individual. It is important to superimpose so that: (a) the changes which it is desired to show are shown, for example, change in mandibular position must not be 'contaminated' by changes in maxillary position; and (b) changes are judged from a relatively unchanging base.

No region of the head can be considered as absolutely stable during growth or treatment, and therefore there is no perfect reference point or line for superimposition. The following considerations have been made in attempts to find reasonable superimposition areas.

1 Since neurocranial growth is largely complete at the end of the seventh year of life, the cranial base is considered to be relatively stable after that time. Growth and treatment change in facial structures are

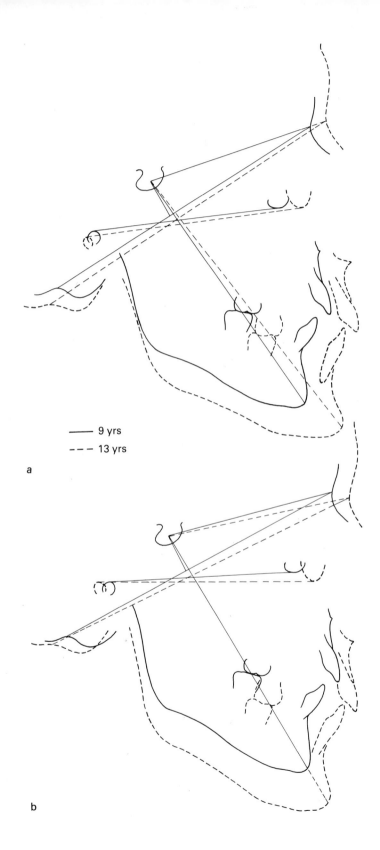

— 9 yrs

--- 13 yrs

a

b

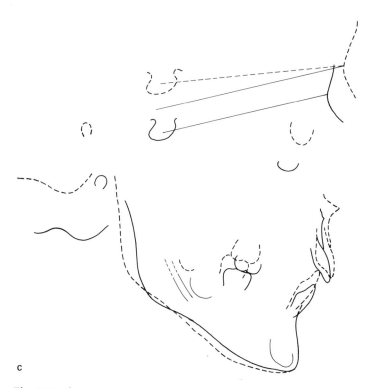

c

Fig. 4.14. The varying effects of different superimposition methods: radiographic outlines (female aged 9 and 13 years). Superimposed on (a) the SN line at S and on (b) the Y-axis at S, showing the apparent differences in growth changes. Superimposition on Björk's mandibular reference structures (c) shows the periosteal remodelling of the mandible and the total mandibular growth rotation in relation to the anterior cranial base (SN line), the degree of rotation being the angle between the SN lines at the two ages.

therefore often related to the anterior cranial base, either by superimposing on De Coster's line and the anterior border of sella turcica or on the sella–nasion line and sella point. The Bolton line broadly averages the slopes of the anterior and middle cranial fossae, and a registration point has been described (Broadbent 1931), which is the mid-point of a perpendicular from sella to the Bolton line. Superimpositions are made on the registration point, with Bolton lines parallel.

2 Björk (1964, 1966), studying growth of maxilla and mandible by means of successional radiographs with metallic implants in the jaws, has suggested that there are certain natural reference structures within the jaws themselves. In the mandible, the natural reference structures are: (a) the anterior border of the symphysis; (b) the endosteal lower border of the symphysis; (c) the trabeculae related to the mandibular canal; and (d) the lower border of a developing molar germ until the roots begin to form. Superimposition is carried out by superimposing on the most anterior structure, the anterior border of the symphysis, and finding a 'best fit' of the other structures.

In the maxilla, the only stable reference structure proposed by Björk is the anterior contour of the zygomatic process. Superimposition on the maxilla is therefore less satisfactory.

The purpose of superimposing on intra-jaw structures is to reveal growth and treatment changes within the jaws themselves, both in the shape of the jaw and in the position of the teeth. Furthermore, by relating the intra-jaw reference structures to an otuside reference line such as the sella–nasion line, angular changes in the body of the jaws, usually known as growth rotation, can be revealed (Björk & Skeiller 1983; Solow & Houston 1988).

3 The sella–gnathion line or Y axis has been considered to be the general line of translatory facial growth, and is sometimes used for superimposition, with sella as the superimposition point.

4 The Frankfort line is, by definition, the horizontal line of the head. If this definition is accepted, this line could be used to orient successive radiographs. It is sometimes used in this way, with sella or registration point being the superimposition point and the Frankfort lines being paralleled. The difficulty of landmark location makes the Frankfort line less than satisfactory for superimposition. An alternative would be to use a true horizontal derived from a radiograph taken with the head in a natural head posture (see below).

The different results obtained by different superimposition methods are shown in Fig. 4.14.

At the present time most clinicians and investigators use cranial base structures for superimposition to show general translatory changes in the jaws during growth and treatment, and Björk's stable reference structures, particularly in the mandible, to show intra-jaw changes of shape and tooth position, and jaw rotation.

In the light of present knowledge it seems that no system of superimposition is substantially better or more accurate than others. Houston and Lee (1985) have reported appreciable errors in several methods of superimposition on cranial base structures, and Cook and Gravely (1988) have reported errors in location of Björk's reference structures. Cook and Southall (1989) also reported substantial errors in several methods of superimposing mandibular outlines, with those using Björk's structures being the least reliable. The accuracy of point location and of superimposition is probably of greater importance than the superimposition method chosen, and it must always be remembered that any changes shown are only the changes related to the chosen superimposition area.

Currently, superimposition is frequently carried out by means of computer plotting and graphics.

Cephalometric assessment in orthodontic diagnosis

The most widespread use of cephalometric assessment is in orthodontic diagnosis, and many systems of assessment have been developed. While these systems differ in detail, they all contain certain basic principles, which will be outlined.

Relationship of upper and lower jaws in the sagittal plane

Since the relationship of the jaws profoundly affects the relationships of the dentition, all orthodontic cephalometric assessments include this feature. It can be assessed in two ways:

(a) Relationship of each jaw to an outside structure. The relationship of each jaw to the anterior cranial base, usually to the sella–nasion line, gives a measurement not only of the position of each jaw but also of the relationship of the jaws to each other. The commonest system is to use the angles SNA and SNB, a method based on the work of Reidel (1952).

The angles SNA and SNB respectively give a measure of the relative positions of maxilla and mandible compared to the anterior cranial base. The accepted ideal angle for SNA is around 80°, and for SNB around 77°. Variation from these angles would indicate variation in maxillary or mandibular position.

The relationship between the two angles SNA and SNB gives a measure of skeletal relationship. When angle SNA is approximately 80°, the ideal skeletal relationship (Class 1) exists when angle SNB is 2° to 4° smaller than angle SNA. When angle SNB is more than 4° smaller than angle SNA a skeletal Class 2 relationship exists, and when angle SNB is less than 2° smaller than angle SNA a skeletal Class 3 relationship exists (Fig. 4.15). Obviously, the greater the discrepancy between angles SNA and SNB the greater the degree of skeletal Class 2 or Class 3 relationship.

This method of assessment of the skeletal relationship has been criticized on the grounds that A and B points do not necessarily represent the true position of the dental bases, and that these points may

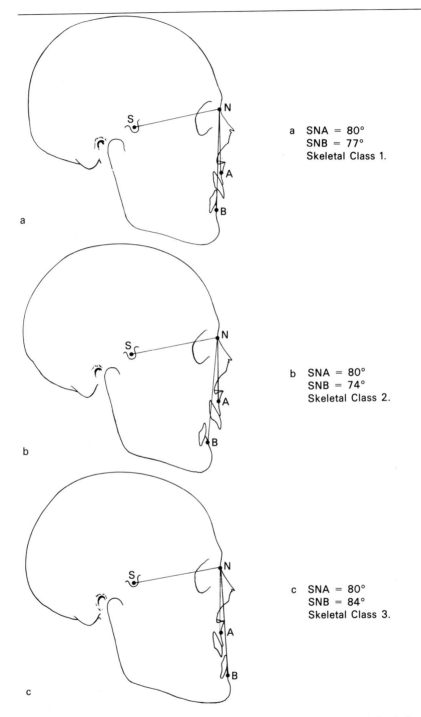

a   SNA = 80°
    SNB = 77°
    Skeletal Class 1.

b   SNA = 80°
    SNB = 74°
    Skeletal Class 2.

c   SNA = 80°
    SNB = 84°
    Skeletal Class 3.

Fig. 4.15. Assessment of skeletal relationship by SNA–SNB difference. (a) Skeletal Class 1, the SNA–SNB difference falls within the range of 2°–4°. (b) Skeletal Class 2, the SNA–SNB difference is greater than 4°. (c) Skeletal Class 3, the SNA–SNB difference is less than 2°.

vary with growth. However, the angles SNA and SNB do give a measure of the degree of prognathism or retrognathism of each jaw at any one time. It must be appreciated that this method of comparison between the two angles becomes invalid if angle SNA deviates markedly from 80°, because the general slope of the upper face would then be different, and the SNA–SNB angular differences would not have the same significance (Fig. 4.16). This can to some extent be overcome by subtracting 0.5° from the SNA–SNB difference for every 1° the SNA measurement is above 80°, and vice versa.

It has also been pointed out (Jarvinen 1980) that the position of S point is variable, and therefore variation in angles SNA and SNB are not necessarily due to variation in jaw position.

(b) Relationship of the jaws to each other. Two main methods exist for assessing the sagittal relationship of the jaws without consideration of outside structures, the method of Ballard (1948) and the 'Wits' analysis (Jacobson 1975, 1988).

The method devised by Ballard (1948) is similar in principle to the clinical method of residual overjet previously described, but it involves actual measurements rather than clinical judgement. It only relates the

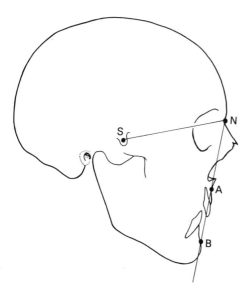

Fig. 4.16. The greater the deviation of angle SNA from 80°, the less valid the method of SNA–SNB difference becomes for assessment of the skeletal relationship. In the illustration, an obvious skeletal Class 2 has an SNA–SNB difference of 0° due to the backward slope of the upper face.

jaws to each other, and does not measure the relationship of each jaw to any outside structure, but it is useful in that it involves a consideration of the inclination of the incisor teeth and a measurement of incisal overjet.

This method is based on the assumptions that:

1   There is an 'ideal' angulation of the upper incisor teeth to the horizontal.

2   There is an 'ideal' inter-incisal angle.

3   The teeth may tilt into their final positions as they erupt, with their pivot point about one third of the root length from the apex.

The outlines of the upper and lower incisor teeth are traced from the lateral radiograph and the long axes of these teeth are drawn from incisal tip to root apex. A pivot point is marked on each long axis one third of the root length from the apex. The outline of the upper incisor is then redrawn on a new long axis angulated at the ideal angle to the maxillary line and passing through the pivot point. The 'ideal' angulation of the upper incisor teeth is generally accepted as about 108° to the maxillary line. A new long axis for the lower incisor is then redrawn, passing through the lower incisor pivot point and angulated at 135° to the 'ideal' upper incisor long axis, this being the 'ideal' inter-incisal angle. The outline of the lower incisor is redrawn on the new long axis line, with the pivot points superimposed. Finally the incisal overjet is measured with the teeth in their new positions. This 'residual overjet' is taken as a measure of any skeletal discrepancy, since abnormal angulation of the teeth has been corrected.

An excessive overjet will indicate a skeletal Class 2 and a reduced or reversed overjet a skeletal Class 3. Fig. 4.17 illustrates the main features of this method.

The main drawback to this method of assessment is the difficulty of outlining the roots of the incisor teeth to determine the long axis of the teeth, particularly in the lower incisors. Furthermore, the assumption that the teeth have a fixed pivot point may not be correct, and the accepted norms for incisor and mandibular inclinations are also in some doubt, and may not be applicable to different populations.

In contrast to most analyses which use angular measurement of jaw relationships, the Wits analysis (Jacobsen 1975, 1988) uses a linear measurement. The method involves constructing perpendiculars from A and B points to the occlusal line, and measuring the distance along the occlusal line between the points of intersection of the perpendiculars. For the ideal Class 1 skeletal relationship, the intersection of the perpendicular from B point to the occlusal line should lie 1 mm in front

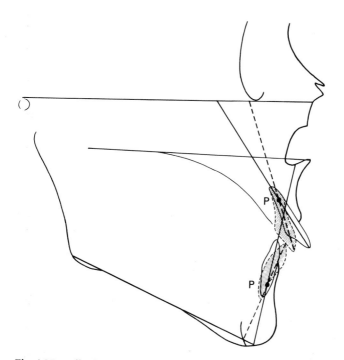

Fig. 4.17. Ballard's method of assessing skeletal relationship. The solid outline represents the actual position the teeth. The dotted outline represents the teeth aligned in their corrected inclinations (shaded), tilted about the pivot points (P). The residual overjet is approximately correct, indicating skeletal Class 1.

of that from A point in males, and the two intersections should coincide in females. For Class 2 and Class 3 skeletal relationships the B point perpendicular intersection will lie further back or further forward respectively, by a measurable amount directly related to the skeletal discrepancy. This method has the virtue of simplicity, but has the drawback that the results vary not only with the skeletal relationship but also with the slope of the occlusal line, which itself does not have a fixed relationship either with other facial lines or with the horizontal.

The measurement of incisal angulations and relationships

Almost all cephalometric diagnostic assessments include measurements of incisal relationships. Generally the long axes of the most prominent upper and lower incisors from the incisal tip to the root apex is drawn, and produced to meet a reference line from which incisal angulations can be measured. Incisal overbite and overjet and the interincisal angle can also be measured. The reference lines used are commonly the sella–nasion line, the Frankfort line and the maxillary line for the upper incisors and the mandibular line for the lower incisors. However, these reference lines are themselves variable when compared with each other and with a true horizontal (Foster *et al.* 1981) and incisal angulations measured in this way should be interpreted with caution. A further possible source of error lies in the difficulty of locating the position of the incisor apices, particularly in the lower jaw.

The measurement of vertical skeletal relationships

A lateral skull radiograph gives the facility to measure not only sagittal but also vertical relationships, and many assessments include such measurements. One of the commonest linear measurements is the measurement of face height, either in total, for example the distance from nasion to menton, or as proportions, for example taking the upper face height as the distance from nasion to ANS and the lower face height from ANS to menton, the face height proportions then being compared. Common angular measurements in the vertical plane relate to the slopes of the occlusal line and of the mandibular line. Both of these are very variable, and are usually measured in relationship to the maxillary, Frankfort or sella–nasion lines. At the extremes of variation the slope of the lower border of the mandible will be reflected in variation in anterior facial height and in incisal overbite.

Using these principles, many systems of diagnostic analysis have been developed. Several of these systems have been reviewed by Brown (1981). It is proposed to outline a simple analysis which will include most of the features mentioned above. The analysis refers to Fig. 4.18.

After location of the appropriate cephalometric points, and construction of the appropriate lines, the following measurements are made:

- *Angle SNA*—maxillary position related to anterior cranial base.
- *Angle SNB*—mandibular position related to anterior cranial base.
- *Angle ANB*—a measure of the skeletal jaw relationship in the sagittal plane.
- *Angle upper incisor to maxillary line (UI–max)*—the relative inclination of the upper incisor
- *Angle lower incisor to mandibular line (LI–mand)*—the relative inclination of the lower incisor
- *Angle upper incisor to lower incisor (UI–LI)*—the interincisal angle
- *Angle maxillary line to mandibular line (MM)*—the relative slope of the lower border of the mandible.

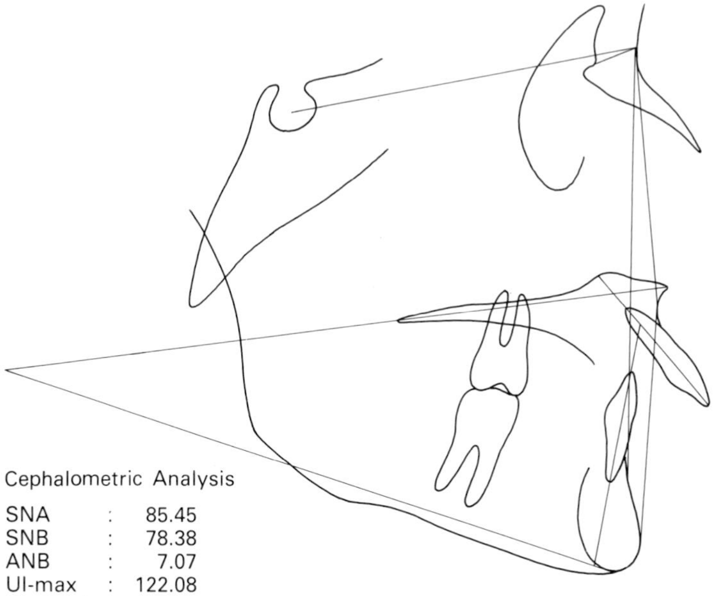

Cephalometric Analysis

SNA	:	85.45
SNB	:	78.38
ANB	:	7.07
UI-max	:	122.08
LI-mand	:	82.86
UI-LI	:	130.00
MM	:	25.07
LI-APO	:	−5.66
LFH	:	53.87
OJ	:	14.61
OB	:	9.69

Fig. 4.18. A cephalometric tracing and measurements. See text for analysis.

- *Distance of lower incisor tip to A–pogonion line (LI–APo)*—a measure of the sagittal relationship of the lower incisor to the jaws.
- *Face height proportions*—usually expressed as the proportion of lower face height (ANS–menton) to total face height (nasion to menton)
- *Incisal overjet*—the horizontal measurement of incisal overlap.
- *Incisal overbite*—the vertical measurement of incisal overlap.

The results of the measurements shown in Fig. 4.18 can be interpreted as follows.

The skeletal relationship is Class 2, of moderate severity (corrected angle ANB is 6°). This can be confirmed with a Ballard's or a Wits analysis. The maxilla is somewhat prognathic in relation to the anterior cranial base (ideal SNA angle is 80°), while the mandibular position is virtually correct (ideal SNB angle is 77°). The upper incisors are markedly proclined, and the lower incisors somewhat retroclined, the interincisal angle being low (ideal UI–LI is 135°). The lower incisors also lie well behind the A–Po line, which reflects their retroclination. The

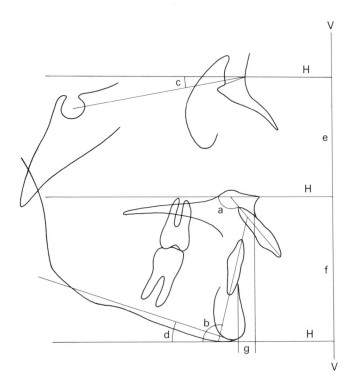

Fig. 4.19. A cephalometric analysis with the radiograph taken in natural head posture. The vertical (V) is recorded on the radiograph by means of a plumb-line. True horizontals (H) are drawn through nasion, ANS and menton. The angulation of upper and lower incisors (a, b), the SN line (c) the mandibular line (d) and any other dento-facial structures can be measured in relation to the horizontal. Face height proportions can be measured as the vertical distance between the three horizontals (e, f). The sagittal skeletal relationship can be measured as the distance between perpendiculars from A and B points to the horizontal line (g).

slope of the mandibular line is almost correct (ideal MM angle is 27°). The occlusal problem thus relates mainly to a forward position of the maxilla with consequent Class 2 occlusal relationship, and modification of the inclination and relationship of the incisors, the latter probably being associated with aberrant lip function consequent on the skeletal discrepancy (see Chapter 5).

The use of natural head posture

It will be appreciated from the foregoing descriptions that cephalometric analysis in orthodontic diagnosis involves the measurement of relationships of various components of the face and jaws to other reference structures. This would be entirely logical if those reference structures were themselves fixed in their spatial relationship, but unfortunately they are not. It has been shown (Foster *et al.* 1981) that the SN, Frankfort, maxillary and mandibular lines, all commonly used for reference, bear no fixed relationship to each other nor to the true horizontal. Furthermore, the range of variation is wide. A more logical approach would be to take the cephalometric radiograph with the head in its natural upright posture, and to derive from that a true horizontal and vertical to which all the facial and jaw structures could be related. Such an analysis is shown in Fig. 4.19. The main drawback to this method is the difficulty of reproducing a natural head posture for every radiograph. Several authors have reported on methods of reproducing natural head posture (Solow & Tallgren 1971; Showfety *et al.* 1983; Cooke & Wei 1988a, 1988b; Sandham 1988), and it seems that with careful attention to the positioning technique the errors in relating the head to the true horizontal are appreciably less than the range of variation of the accepted reference lines. Since this approach to analysis is more logical, even though more demanding of careful radiographic technique, it is likely that it will become more widely used.

Cephalometric assessment in treatment planning

Just as cephalometric assessments are widely used in diagnosis, so they can be used in the planning of orthodontic treatment. The Ricketts analysis (1972) includes an analysis of dento-facial form, a prediction of growth changes and a 'visualized treatment objective', in which the final tooth and jaw positions to be aimed for by treatment in conjunction with growth are plotted and drawn over the lateral skull radiograph. More simple methods which do not include growth predictions are also in common use, and the prognosis for any type of tooth movement in the sagittal plane can readily be plotted on a radiograph. As an example, a prognosis assessment for simple treatment in Class 2 Division 1 incisor relationship involving only tipping movements of upper incisors and overbite reduction will be described (Fig. 4.20).

Simple prognosis assessment

The outlines of a lateral skull radiograph are traced, to include the outlines of the upper and lower incisors and of the soft tissue profile of the face. The long axes of the incisor teeth are added and the pivot point

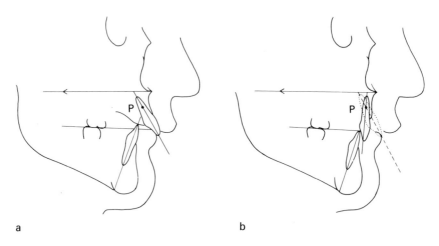

a   b

Fig. 4.20. Prognosis tracing for simple treatment of a Class 2 Division 1 occlusion, involving overbite reduction and tipping of upper incisors. (a) The original tracing, showing the excessive overbite, proclined upper incisors and lip trap. (b) The prognosis tracing, showing the overbite reduction to the level of the occlusal line, and the tipping back of the upper incisors to a correct overjet relationship. In this case the new upper incisal angle (85°) and interincisal angle (170°) are outside the acceptable limits of stability. Such simple treatment would probably therefore not be successful.

of the upper incisor is marked, one third of the root length from the apex. The maxillary line and the occlusal line are also marked on the tracing. On a superimposed tracing the bony and soft tissue outlines are drawn and the same pivot point is marked. The lower incisor outline is then redrawn on the same long axis but with the incisal edge at the level of the occlusal line. The reduction of the overbite to this extent is relatively simple treatment (see Chapter 13). The upper incisor outline is then redrawn in such a position that the overjet is reduced to normal, while the pivot points coincide. This represents simple tipping of the upper incisors to their new position. The superimposed tracing will then have the original facial outlines and the new incisor positions. To decide whether such simple treatment is realistic it is necessary to measure the new angulation of the upper incisors and the new inter-incisal angle. An acceptable range some 10° either side of the ideal might be considered a reasonable compromise. Any result outside this range would probably not be functionally stable. It is also necessary to consider whether the overbite reduction would be sufficient, and this can be visualized on the tracing. Finally the soft tissue relationships to the teeth in their new position can be seen on the superimposed tracing.

For an assessment of prognosis for such simple treatment of a Class 3 incisor relationship the final judgement of feasibility would need to be made using the other end of the range of acceptable compromise angulations of the teeth, and there would need to be a positive incisal overbite for stability.

If the final judgement showed the angulation of the teeth to be outside the acceptable range, then a plan would need to be made incorporating more complex tooth movements, which could also be drawn on a prognosis tracing.

Variation in the skeletal relationship

Normal variation in the skeletal relationship exists in all populations. As mentioned in Chapter 1, it was previously thought to be largely environmental in nature, the total growth of the jaws being related to nutrition, masticatory function and the presence or absence of upper respiratory infection. It is fairly generally accepted at present that the form and relationship of the jaws is much more dependent on inherited factors, with the functional aspects which contribute to normal jaw growth also being to a large extent genetically determined. The broad racial variations in skeletal relationship have been described in Chapter 1. The individual variation within populations is wide ranging, from extremes of Class 3 relationship to extremes of Class 2 relationship (see Fig. 4.3). It is likely that various populations differ in the proportions of the different skeletal patterns which they contain. This to a large extent depends on population movements and mixtures. There may be local differences within one country, and with more population movements occurring it becomes increasingly more unrealistic to define a 'typical' face for any particular area.

Foster and Day (1974) in a study of Shropshire children aged 11−12 years, found the following distribution of skeletal relationships.

Skeletal Class 1	40.8%
Skeletal Class 2	53.8%
Skeletal Class 3	5.3%

From this it can be seen that, in some populations at least, Class 2 relationship is more 'normal' than the ideal Class 1 relationship.

Change in skeletal relationship with growth

Although the relationship of the jaws is largely genetically determined, it is incorrect to regard it as immutable. Differential growth of the jaws can and sometimes does produce change in the skeletal pattern. In particular the puberal growth spurt may affect one jaw more than the other, producing changes which sometimes help and sometimes hinder orthodontic treatment. It has been shown, by means of growth studies, that maxillary or mandibular prognathism may increase or decrease during growth, with consequent change in the antero-posterior relationship of the jaws and of the dental arches.

Summary

Factors affecting occlusal development

1   General factors

- Skeletal factors of the jaws.
- Muscular environment of the teeth.
- Size of the dentition in relation to size of the jaws.

2   Local factors

- Aberrant developmental position of teeth.
- Supernumerary teeth.
- Hypodontia.
- Effects of certain habits.
- Localized soft tissue anomalies.

Skeletal factors

Jaw size, form and relationship affects the final position of the teeth, and limits orthodontic treatment.

Skeletal relationship (skeletal pattern, dental base relationship) is the antero-posterior relationship of the basal parts of the jaws to each other in occlusion.

Variation in skeletal relationship may result from variation in size and/or in position of the jaws.

Lateral and vertical relationships are also important.

Alveolar bone and tooth relationship may be different from skeletal relationship.

Methods of assessment of skeletal relationship

1 Clinical

- Visual
- Palpation
- Method of residual overjet

2 Radiological

- Using standardized lateral skull radiographs

The use of cephalometrics in orthodontics

1 Superimposition of radiographs in growth and treatment studies.
2 Orthodontic diagnosis:
    - using intra-cranial reference lines;
    - using natural head posture.
3 Treatment planning and prognosis.

Skeletal relationship is largely genetically determined. Differences in pattern of variation exist in different populations. Growth changes are possible in skeletal relationship.

References

Ballard, C. F. (1948) Some bases for aetiology and diagnosis in orthodontics. *Dent Rec*, **68**, 133–145.

Björk, A. (1966) Sutural growth of the upper face studied by the implant method. *Acta Odontol Scand*, **24**, 109–127.

Björk, A., Krebs, A. & Solow, B. (1964) A method for epidemiological registration of malocclusion. *Acta Odontol Scand*, **22**, 27–41.

Björk, A. & Skeiller, V. (1983) Normal and abnormal growth of the mandible: a synthesis of longitudinal cephalometric implant studies over a period of 25 years. *Eur J. Orthod*, **5**, 1–46.

Broadbent, B. H. (1931) A new X-ray technique and its application to orthodontics. *Angle Orthod*, **1**, 45–66.

Brown, M. (1981) Eight methods of analysing a cephalogram to establish antero-posterior skeletal discrepancy. *Br J Orthod*, **8**, 139–146.

Cook, P. A. & Gravely, J. F. (1988) Tracing error with Björk's mandibular structures. *Angle Orthod*, **58**, 169–178.

Cook, P. A. & Southall, P. J. (1989) The reliability of mandibular radiographic superimposition. *Br J Orthod*, **16**, 25–30.

Cooke, M. S. & Wei, S. H. Y. (1988a) A summary five-factor cephalometric analysis based on natural head posture and the true horizontal. *Am J Orthod*, **93**, 213–223.

Cooke, M. S. & Wei, S. H. Y. (1988b) An improved method for the assessment of the sagittal skeletal pattern and its correlation to previous methods. *Eur J Orthod,* **10,** 122–127.

De Coster, L. (1952) The familial line, studied by a new line of reference. *Trans Eur Orthod Soc,* **28,** 50–55.

Foster, T. D. & Day, A. J. W. (1974) A survey of malocclusion and the need for orthodontic treatment in a Shropshire school population. *Br J Orthod,* **1,** 73–78.

Foster, T. D., Howat, A. P. & Naish, P. J. (1981) Variation in cephalometric reference lines. *Br J Orthod,* **8,** 183–187.

Holdaway, R. A. (1983) A soft tissue cephalometric analysis and its use in orthodontic treatment planning. *Am J Orthod,* **84,** 1–28.

Houston, W. J. B. & Lee, R. T. (1985) Accuracy of different methods of radiographic superimposition on cranial base structures. *Eur J Orthod,* **7,** 127–135.

Jacobson, A. (1975) The 'Wits' appraisal of jaw disharmony. *Am J Orthod,* **67,** 125–133.

Jacobson, A. (1988) Update on the Wits analysis. *Angle Orthod,* **58,** 205–219.

Jarvinen, S. (1980) Relation of SNA angle to saddle angle. *Am J Orthod,* **78,** 670–673.

Ricketts, R. M. (1957) Planning treatment on the basis of the facial pattern and an estimate of its growth. *Angle Orthod,* **27,** 14–37.

Ricketts, R. M. (1972) The value of cephalometrics in computerised technology. *Angle Orthod,* **42,** 179–199.

Riedel, R. R. (1952) The relation of maxillary structures to cranium in malocclusion and in normal occlusion. *Angle Orthod,* **22,** 142–145.

Sandham, J. A. (1988) Repeatability of head posture recordings from lateral cephalometric radiographs. *Br J Orthod,* **15,** 157–162.

Showfety, K. J., Vig, P. S. & Matteson, S. (1983) A simple method for taking natural head posture cephalograms. *Am J Orthod,* **83,** 495–500.

Solow, B. & Houston W. J. B. (1988) Mandibular growth rotations—their mechanisms and importance. *Eur J Orthod,* **10,** 369–373.

Solow, B. & Tallgren, A. (1971) Natural head position in standing subjects. *Acta Odontol Scand,* **29,** 591–607.

Williams, R. (1969) The diagnostic line. *Am J Orthod,* **55,** 458–476.

5

Muscle factors affecting occlusal development

The teeth erupt into an environment of functional activity governed by the muscles of mastication, of the tongue and of the face. The muscles of the tongue, lips and cheeks are of particular importance in guiding the teeth into their final position, and variation in muscle form and function can affect the position and occlusion of the teeth. It must be remembered that all muscles exert their influence by virtue of the site of their origins and insertions. The muscles of the lips, cheeks and tongue have their main origins on the basal parts of the jaws, and therefore the position of the jaws must affect the position and action of the muscles which function on the teeth. It is thus not realistic to consider the muscles in isolation without reference to the bony structures with which they interrelate in guiding the erupting teeth.

The lips

The several muscles making up the lips can conveniently be considered as a single functional unit, since that is the way in which they normally work. They play their part in occlusal development by virtue of their size, form and function. The form and function of the lips can be considered in two planes, vertical and sagittal.

Vertical form of the lips

In the ideal lip form, the vertical dimension is such that, with the lip muscles in their position of resting posture, the lips meet together (Fig. 5.1a). In this condition of rest, there is minimal muscle contraction to maintain the position of the lips, and therefore minimal electrical action potential is detectable by electromyography. For this reason it has been called the position of 'electrical silence', though this is not strictly correct.

Considerable variation occurs in the resting lip form. In many individuals the lips do not meet in the rest position, a condition sometimes referred to as 'lip incompetence', and in some the space between the lips at rest is very pronounced (Fig. 5.1b). The reason for the discrepancy may be in the shape of the jaws, for example, when a high mandibular gonial angle places the origin of the lower lip too far

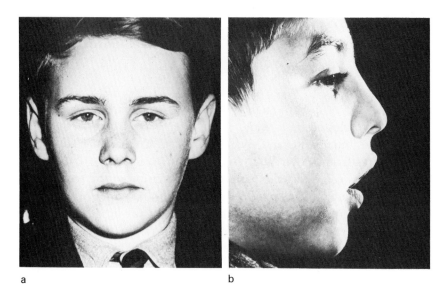

a   b

Fig. 5.1. Variation in the form of the lips in the vertical dimension. (a) The lips are of sufficient size to meet at rest. (b) Vertical lip incompetence. At rest the lips are apart.

down in relation to the upper lip. In most cases, however, the source of the discrepancy lies in the lips themselves, which may simply be too short in the vertical dimension, or the wrong shape to meet at rest.

The importance of discrepancies in vertical size or form of the lips lies in the fact that the lips are usually brought together during swallowing and speech movements. If they are of sufficient size to be together at rest then lip closure will not place extra forces on the teeth. If the lips at rest are apart, then muscular contraction will be required to bring them together during swallowing and speech, and such contraction will impose extra forces on the erupting teeth. Furthermore, some people, whose lips do not meet at rest, maintain a conscious lip closure for much of the time, again imposing muscular forces on the teeth. The effect of these forces on the erupting teeth depends to a large extent on the sagittal relationship of the lips.

Sagittal relationship of the lips

The sagittal relationship of the lips is almost entirely determined by the relationship of the basal bone of the jaws, to which they are attached. The lower lip tends to be further back than the upper lip in a skeletal Class 2 relationship, and further forward in a skeletal Class 3 relationship (Fig. 5.2). This not only increases the difficulty of putting

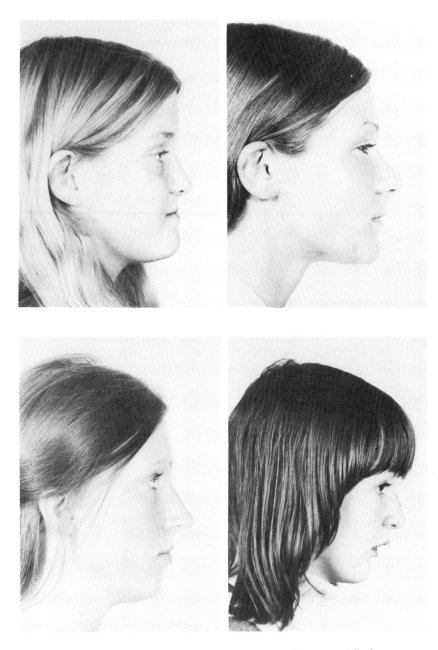

Fig. 5.2. Variation in lip position in the sagittal dimension. This is essentially due to variation in basal bone relationship.

the lips together, but also may cause the lower lip to modify the eruptive path of the upper incisors. Such modification may alter the primary effect of the skeletal relationship on the occlusal relationship of the teeth, either increasing or reducing the effect of any skeletal discrepancy. For example, with a skeletal Class 2 relationship the lower lip may function completely or partly behind the upper incisors. If the skeletal discrepancy is not severe, the lip may procline the upper incisors so that the occlusal relationship is more severely Class 2 than the skeletal relationship (Fig. 5.3a). If the skeletal discrepancy is severe, the lower lip may function behind the upper incisors without causing them to be proclined (Fig. 5.3b). In other instances, with skeletal Class 2, the lower lip functions entirely in front of the upper incisors, causing them to be retroclined into the Class 2 Division 2 incisor relationship (Fig. 5.4). It is equally possible for lip activity to produce Class 2 or Class 3 occlusal relationships on a Class 1 skeletal relationship by altering the inclination of the incisor teeth during eruption or to produce Class 1 occlusion on Class 2 or Class 3 skeletal relationship if the skeletal discrepancy is not severe.

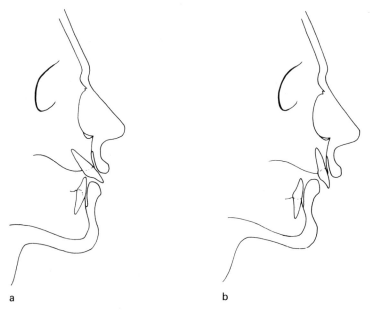

a   b

Fig. 5.3. The effect of skeletal relationship on lip function and incisor position. (a) In a mild skeletal Class 2 the lower lip may procline the upper incisors. (b) In a more severe skeletal Class 2 the lower lip can function behind the upper incisors without causing proclination.

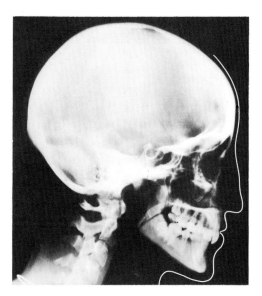

Fig. 5.4. Skeletal Class 2 relationship, with the lower lip functioning in front of the upper incisors causing incisor retroclination and a Class 2 Division 2 incisor relationship.

In modifying the inclination of incisor teeth during eruption, the lips often act in conjunction with the effects of tongue function, thumb sucking habits or crowding of the teeth.

Function of the lips

Apart from lip functions mentioned above, other activity of the lips can modify erupting tooth positions. The lower lip plays more part than the upper lip both in functional movements and in governing the position of the incisor teeth. The lower lip may cause retroclination of the lower incisors in normal function during swallowing, speech and smiling activities (Fig. 5.5). Thus the ultimate position of the incisor teeth, both before and after any orthodontic treatment, is very much dependent on lip activity.

The lip-line

The level at which the lips meet together in normal function is usually called the 'lip-line'. The position of the lip-line in relation to the incisor teeth plays a part in governing the position of those teeth. The ideal level of the lip-line is approximately at the centre of the crowns of the upper incisor teeth, with the lower lip in front of the upper incisors (Fig. 5.6a). The lip-line may be low, in which case part of the lower lip may function

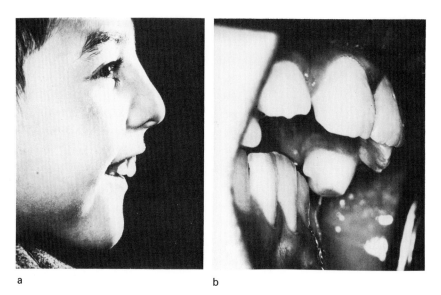

a   b

Fig. 5.5. Functional activity of the lower lip. (a) Retraction of the lower lip across the lower incisors during normal function may cause (b) retroclination of the lower incisors and excessive overjet.

behind the upper incisors, causing proclination (Fig. 5.6.). If the lower lip functions completely behind the upper incisors the definition of lip-line is not strictly applicable (Fig. 5.6c). The lip-line may be high, as is common in Class 2 Division 2 occlusal relationship. This is usually brought about by the fact that retroclination of the incisors results in the incisors not meeting correctly, with consequent continued development of upper and lower incisors and related alveolar bone in the vertical dimension. The upper incisors are thus too far down in relation to the lips, and the lip-line is high (Fig. 5.6d).

The tongue

The tongue, functioning mainly in conjunction with the lips and cheeks, is the other major guiding force for the erupting teeth. The extrinsic muscles of the tongue are attached to the inner aspects of the mandible, the hyoid bone, the palate and the styloid process. It therefore lies within the arch of the lower jaw, and affects the developing teeth by virtue of its size, its resting posture and its function.

Tongue size in relation to the size of the lower jaw is rarely at fault, but occasionally, if the lower jaw is larger than the upper jaw, the tongue is too large to fit within the upper dental arch. In such cases the

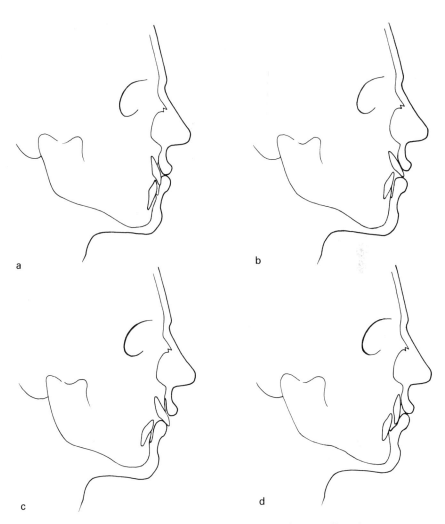

Fig. 5.6. Variation in lip-line. (a) The ideal level, the lower lip controlling the upper incisors. (b) A low lip-line, the lower lip functioning partly behind the upper incisors. (c) The lower lip functioning completely behind the upper incisors. (d) A high lip-line, the lower lip exerting extra control over the upper incisors, which are retroclined.

tongue usually finds space between the upper and lower arches and prevents the full vertical development of the dento-alveolar structures resulting in open bite of varying extent.

The resting position of the tongue is ideally completely within the dental arches, filling the space enclosed by the teeth. Sometimes, however, the tongue takes up an adaptive postural position, slightly protruded between the teeth to touch the lower lip. It has been suggested that this adaptive position of the tongue is produced in order to seal the front of the mouth to allow nasal breathing, when there is difficulty in holding the lips together due to vertical or sagittal lip discrepancy. It may be combined with an adaptive forward postural position of the mandible. The adaptive tongue position between the incisor teeth may prevent full vertical development of the incisal segments, and consequently may produce an incomplete overbite, or more severely an anterior open bite (Fig. 5.7).

The muscular function of the tongue is particularly concerned with

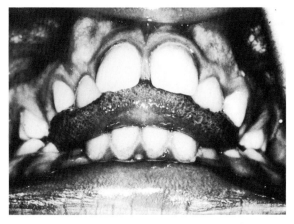

a

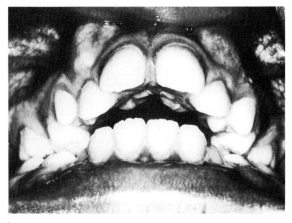

b

Fig. 5.7. Adaptive postural position of the tongue. (a) The tongue rests between the upper and lower incisors to maintain contact with the lower lip. (b) Full vertical development of the incisal segment is prevented, and there is an incomplete overbite.

mastication, swallowing and speech. Its effect on the developing dentition can most readily be studied with regard to swallowing function. In the voluntary phase of swallowing, after mastication is complete the food is collected on the dorsal surface of the tongue by the action of the tongue and the facial muscles. The lips are then closed, and the teeth brought into light occlusal contact. The tongue is elevated into the palate and the muscular action of the tongue and the floor of the mouth pushes the food back into the pharynx, this action being accompanied by a momentary clenching of the teeth. A similar swallowing activity occurs when swallowing saliva, though fluids in larger quantity are usually swallowed with the lips and teeth apart. The essential features of normal swallowing of solid food and saliva, are:

1 Closure of the lips.
2 Teeth in light occlusal contact.
3 Tongue elevated to the palate.
4 Momentary clenching of the teeth as food passes into the pharynx.

Many variations of normal swallowing activity are seen, and there is no complete agreement regarding the nature and origin of these variations. Furthermore, the effects of these variations on the developing occlusion are themselves not constant. In the light of current knowledge and experience, two main patterns of variation could be described, although there is often difficulty in distinguishing between the two. Neither of these variations appears to be common, and at present they are not fully understood. They may be described as follows.

Adaptive swallowing

Adaptive swallowing involves the positioning of the tongue between the teeth during swallowing, and may be carried out with the buccal teeth apart or together.

Tooth apart adaptive swallowing

In swallowing with the buccal teeth apart, the tongue is positioned between the teeth and therefore does not fill the upper arch. Pressures, both muscle and air pressures, within the upper arch are therefore reduced, and this may lead to narrowing of the arch and the production of buccal crossbite, usually unilateral crossbite. Full vertical development of the anterior dento-alveolar segments may be prevented by the tongue, leading to incomplete overbite.

Tooth together adaptive swallowing

The adaptive swallowing with the buccal teeth together involves the forward positioning of the tongue between the incisor teeth during swallowing. This usually results in production of an incomplete overbite or anterior open bite.

Various theories have been put forward to explain adaptive swallowing. Perhaps the most commonly held view is that the forward tongue position is an adaptation to form an anterior oral seal during swallowing, as with an adaptive postural position of the mandible. Its main importance in orthodontic assessment and treatment is that, although it modifies the position of the teeth, it will change with growth or when teeth are re-positioned by treatment, and is therefore not an immutable barrier to orthodontic treatment.

Swallowing with endogenous tongue thrust

In a small proportion of subjects the swallowing activity is accompanied by an anterior thrust of the tongue which appears to be a basic neuromuscular mechanism. This so-called 'endogenous' tongue thrust is sometimes associated with an anterior lisp during speech. It usually affects the developing teeth to the extent of preventing the full vertical development of the anterior dento-alveolar segments, so that an incomplete overbite or, more usually, an anterior open bite, develops. The upper and lower incisors may be proclined by the action of the tongue (Fig. 5.8), though sometimes the lower incisors are retroclined by the contraction of the lower lip during swallowing (Fig. 5.9). Occasionally this type of swallowing activity appears to have no adverse effect on the developing occlusion.

The endogenous tongue thrust is fortunately not common, appearing in only 3.1% of the population studied by Foster and Day (1974). If it is a normal neuromuscular mechanism rather than an adaptive or habit activity, it would not be modified by orthodontic treatment. Re-positioning the teeth would not be likely to alter the tongue activity, and any open bite caused by the tongue thrust would be likely to recur.

It can be seen from this description that these two variations on normal swallowing activity often appear to have somewhat similar effects on the developing occlusion, but, if we accept the essential difference in their nature, they respond differently to orthodontic treatment designed to reposition the teeth. The 'adaptive' tongue activity will change if the teeth are moved so that the adaptation becomes unnecessary, but the 'endogenous' tongue thrust will not

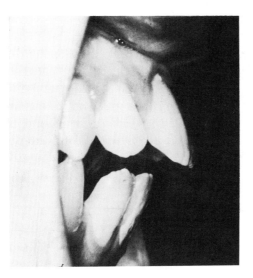

Fig. 5.8. Proclination of upper and lower incisors, and anterior open bite, resulting from tongue-thrusting activity.

change, and will reproduce original tooth positions if these are altered. It is obviously desirable, therefore, to be able to distinguish between the two when planning orthodontic treatment. Unfortunately, it is not always possible to make a clear distinction, particularly from a single clinical assessment. A tongue thrust associated with a noticeable lisp and a wide anterior open bite may reasonably be assumed to be of the

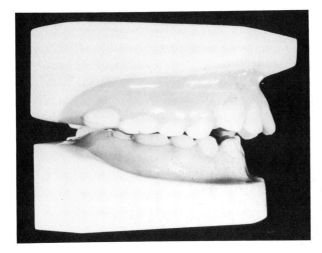

Fig. 5.9. Proclination of upper incisors, and anterior open bite due to tongue thrusting. The lower lip contraction has produced retroclination of the lower incisors.

'endogenous' type, particularly if a parent has the same condition, though such a diagnosis should not be made in a young child, who may simply be going through a normal phase of speech development. There are, in fact, no established criteria for distinguishing between the variations in tongue activity, and more research is needed on this aspect of the oral environment. In the meanwhile assessments are usually made on a 'clinical judgement' or on a trial and error basis, and it must be realized that treatment to correct tooth malpositions caused by tongue activity will not always be successful.

Occlusal development and speech

As speech production involves muscular activity of the tongue it is tempting to speculate either that the position of the teeth may affect speech or that speech activity may affect tooth position. There is no good evidence that either of these alternatives is correct. Normal speech can take place in the presence of severe tooth malposition, and indeed it has been shown that even the fitting of orthodontic appliances has only transient effects on normal speech. Equally, severe articulatory speech defects can occur in the presence of ideal occlusion and position of the teeth. Speech is a complex process involving innate neuromuscular behaviour patterns reinforced by kinesthetic and auditory feedback mechanisms. There appear to be certain circumstances in which neuro-muscular behaviour affects both the speech and the position of the teeth, for example where tongue activity produces an anterior open bite and a lisp, but in such a case it can hardly be said that the speech affects the tooth position since both are secondary to the muscular behaviour. There may be circumstances in which tooth position affects speech, for example in the grossly distorted dental arches frequently seen in patients with cleft lip and palate, in whom there is a high prevalence of articulatory speech defects, but this is far from certain, and many other causes for the speech defects are possible in such patients. Until more is known about the effects of speech on tooth position and of tooth position on speech it is probably wiser to accept that any relationship between the two is unlikely to be simple cause and effect, but is likely to be influenced by other interrelating factors.

Thumb and finger sucking

Thumb and finger sucking activity is so closely related to the oral musculature that it is convenient to consider it at this point. This activity is so common in young children that it can be considered as normal in infancy, though not necessarily so when prolonged into later childhood. In a study of children at $2\frac{1}{2}$ years of age, the author has found that 33% sucked the thumb or fingers, 32% sucked an artificial comforter and only 35% had never exhibited any habitual non-nutritive sucking.

Larsson (1988) studying a group of Swedish children, found that 50% of those who had a thumb or finger sucking activity in infancy retained the habit to at least 7 years of age.

There is some difference of opinion as to whether digit sucking activity is learned or innate. Usually it starts very early in childhood, being evident within a very short time after birth, and there is evidence to suggest that it may begin before birth, but Ayer (1970) presents evidence supporting the theory that prolonged digit sucking is a learned activity. Bakwin (1971), in a study of monozygotic and dizygotic twins, concluded that there is unlikely to be a genetic basis for finger sucking activity which persists after the third birthday. It may be, therefore, that thumb or finger sucking in early childhood is an innate activity in many children, but that prolongation of the activity after infancy may be the result of learning. In any case, prolonged digit sucking will be present from the beginning of occlusal development, and may modify the position of the teeth.

There are many types of habitual sucking activity, some involving digit sucking, others involving sucking of the tongue or lips. The term 'sucking' in this respect indicates a rhythmic activity akin to suckling, which is the normal method of infant feeding. A reduced intra oral air pressure is created, probably by lowering the mandible and tongue, thus increasing the size of the enclosed oral cavity. Day and Foster (1971) have demonstrated the rhythmic variation in intra oral air pressure during thumb and tongue sucking activity. In some children the tongue is protruded beneath the thumb, so that both thumb and tongue are between the teeth. In others, only the thumb lies between the teeth, and the lower incisors may produce a patch of hardened skin on the back of the thumb.

The effects of sucking habits on occlusal development are variable, and to some extent depend on the actual pattern of the habit activity. Thus thumb sucking may be expected to have a different effect from finger sucking, as in Fig. 5.10. Sometimes no effect can be seen. Most commonly, the presence of the thumb between the erupting teeth causes an anterior open bite, which is usually asymmetrical, being more pronounced on the side on which the thumb is sucked (Fig. 5.11). If the tongue is also protruded, the open bite tends to be larger. There is also

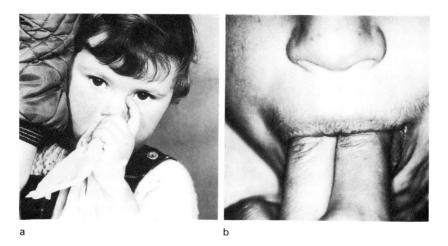

Fig. 5.10. (a) Typical thumb sucking; and (b) finger sucking activity. These two types of sucking habit are likely to have different effects on the developing dentition.

often a unilateral crossbite (Modeer *et al.* 1982). It is thought that the crossbite is brought about by the slight narrowing of the upper dental arch resulting from the reduced intra oral air pressure, possibly combined with the activity of the buccal musculature (Day & Foster 1971). This slight narrowing of the dental arch leads to the lower jaw adopting a translocated path of closure, with development of a crossbite on one side. (See crossbite, Chapter 7).

Thumb and finger sucking habits only really become a problem if they persist into the period of the permanent dentition. It is unlikely that these habits affect the growth of the basal parts of the jaws, their effects being confined to the teeth and the alveolar processes of the jaws. When the habit is stopped, the anterior dento-alveolar segments will usually grow into correct occlusal positions, unless some other factor, such as tongue or lip activity intervenes (Larsson 1972). It is not known whether the unilateral crossbite is self-correcting.

Much time and effort has been expended in attempts to persuade children to give up sucking the thumb or fingers, though the effects of tongue sucking and lip sucking usually go unnoticed. Experience suggests that attempts to stop thumb or finger sucking usually fail unless the child wishes to stop, in which case the fitting of any appliance in the mouth, after appropriate discussion with the child, is usually sufficient to cause the habit to be given up. In practical terms, this usually means delaying any attempt to stop these habits until the age of 8 years or more, by which time, of course, most children will have grown out of the habit.

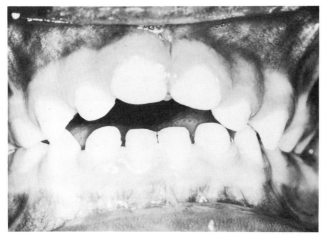

a

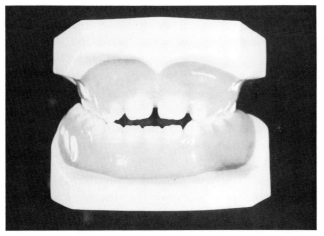

b

Fig. 5.11. The effects of thumb sucking, showing (a) the asymmetry of the anterior open bite, and (b) the unilateral crossbite, which are often seen.

Larsson (1988) reported that significantly more 9-year-old children stopped the thumb or finger sucking habit within 1 year when treated either with verbal encouragement or with an intra-oral appliance than did similar children who received no such treatment.

Dummy sucking

The sucking of a dummy or comforter is usually confined to the first 3 or 4 years of life, being given up, on the whole, sooner than thumb sucking. It produces in most cases some degree of anterior open bite in the primary teeth, unless the hard ring of the dummy is held between the teeth, in which case it can produce other tooth malpositions (Fig. 5.12). Its effects on the developing occlusion seem to be transient.

The neutral zone

Although the teeth erupt into an environment of active muscular forces, and are guided into their occlusal positions by muscle movement, it seems reasonable to believe that, once they have reached their occlusal positions, all the forces acting upon them are equalized to maintain the relatively stable situation which we known as the occlusion. It is well recognized that this is not a position of absolute stability, and that teeth are capable of altering their positions in certain circumstances. Changes take place during growth, and even after growth has ceased minor tooth movements may occur, usually as a result of change in the periodontal supporting structures. Nevertheless, the muscular forces acting directly on the teeth, that is the muscles of the lips, cheeks and tongue, must be in balance if the teeth are to remain in a position of reasonable stability.

The fact that the lips and cheeks function outside and the tongue within the dental arches has led to the concept of a 'neutral zone' existing between the inner and outer perimeters of the dental arches, where the forces of lips and cheeks on the one hand and of the tongue on the other are balanced, and within which the teeth are positioned. This concept of a neutral zone has been challenged by several investigators, largely as a result of measuring the muscle forces on the teeth. Such measurements have shown that the pressures exerted by the lingual musculature appear to exceed those exerted by the perioral musculature. If this is really so, the teeth could not be in a state of balance within the various muscular forces, yet there must be some balance of forces, otherwise the teeth would move. Orthodontic treatment is based on the fact that teeth move under the influence of continuous gentle force.

An explanation of this apparent paradox may be found in the fact that direct muscle forces are not the only forces acting on the teeth.

Moss (1980) has suggested that the equilibrium position of the teeth is dependent on several factors, including forces from the oral musculature, occlusal forces from the muscles of mastication and the integrity of the periodontal ligament.

Air pressure differences can also affect the form of the dental arches. Day and Foster (1971) and Gould and Picton (1975) have demonstrated

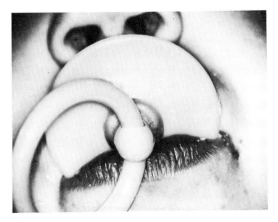

a

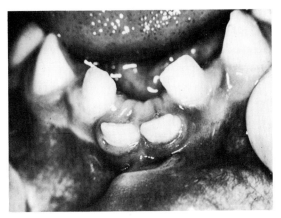

b

Fig. 5.12. Tooth malposition caused by the ring of a comforter being held behind the lower primary central incisors.

sub-atmospheric pressures within the mouth during the normal swallowing process and at rest. The presence of sub-atmospheric pressures may help to explain the findings that direct muscle forces on the lingual side of the arches appear to be greater than on the labial and buccal aspects.

Thus the neutral zone, in which the teeth are in stable position, must be considered not only in relation to muscle forces but also in relation to intraoral air pressures which are induced by mandibular positions and movements, and to occlusal contacts and the periodontal ligament, and in this light the concept of a neutral zone seems reasonable.

As muscle form and function is to a large extent genetically determined, alteration of muscle activity at a subconscious level by education is difficult. The changes most likely to occur are changes in adaptive positions and functions when the need for adaptation is altered. Therefore, not only are the teeth positioned in a neutral zone of the oral environment as a result of development, but they must also be in a neutral zone at the end of any orthodontic treatment, otherwise they will move to take up other positions. This neutral zone has been called a position of 'muscle balance', but, as has been outlined above, it probably involves more than just direct muscle pressures.

Changes in the muscular environment of the teeth during growth

Changes during growth can affect the muscular environment of the teeth as well as the size and relationship of the jaws.

If the lips do not meet at rest there is a tendency for them to remain apart much of the time during childhood, but to be held together by muscular activity progressively more as the child grows up. This puts more pressure on the incisor teeth. There is some evidence that the tongue ceases to grow before the completion of facial development, thus altering the relationship between tongue and jaw size. These factors, together with maturation of muscle activity and force, may be partly responsible for the slight changes in incisor position commonly seen in adolescence and early adult life. The effects of cessation of thumb and finger sucking habits have been mentioned previously, and it seems likely that other rhythmic oral muscular activities may change during growth, with consequent change in tooth position.

It is important, therefore, not to regard the muscular environment of the teeth as having a fixed pattern of activity. Changes can and often do occur, and although the noticeable effects of such changes may be small, they may nevertheless produce alteration in tooth position.

Summary

Final tooth position is largely governed by muscle action, particularly muscles of the lips, cheeks and tongue.

The effect of these muscles is modified by the position of their bony attachments, i.e. by the skeletal relationship.

Lip form is important in the vertical and the sagittal dimension.

Vertical dimension determines the amount of lip pressure on the teeth. Sagittal dimension determines the position of lip pressure on the teeth.

Lip activity may modify the effects of the skeletal relationship on the occlusion of the teeth, particularly by altering the inclination of the erupting incisors.

Tongue size, resting position and *function* can affect the developing occlusion.

Adaptive resting posture or adaptive swallowing may produce incomplete overbite.

'*Endogenous*' tongue thrust may affect incisor positions, and cannot be changed by treatment.

There is a lack of criteria for distinguishing between 'adaptive' and 'endogenous' tongue activity.

The effects of speech on occlusal development and the effects of tooth position on speech are not fully understood, and any apparent effects are likely to be influenced by other interrelated factors.

Thumb and finger sucking, and other sucking activities, may affect the developing occlusion, producing anterior open bite and unilateral cross-bite in some cases. The effect is confined to tooth position, there being little effect on growth of the basal parts of the jaws.

A neutral zone appears to exist within the oral cavity, where the teeth attain a stable position within the muscle forces acting on them and the air pressures induced by those forces.

Re-education of the oral muscles to produce different effects on the teeth is difficult, and the teeth must be in a position of balance between the various forces, both before and after orthodontic treatment.

The muscular environment of the teeth does not have a fixed pattern of activity, but can change during growth, with consequent changes in tooth position.

References

Ayer, W. J. (1970) Psychology and thumbsucking. *J Am Dent Assoc*, **80**, 1335–1337.

Bakwin, H. (1971) Persistent finger sucking in twins. *Dev Med Child Neurol*, **13**, 308–309.

Day, A. J. W. & Foster, T. D. (1971) An investigation into the prevalence of molar crossbite and some associated aetiological conditions. *Dent Practit*, **21**, 402–410.

Foster, T. D. & Day, A. J. W. (1974) A survey of malocclusion and the need for orthodontic treatment in a Shropshire school population. *Br J Orthod* , **1**, 73–78.

Gould, M. S. E. & Picton, D. C. A. (1975) Sub atmospheric pressures and forces recorded from the labiobuccal surfaces of teeth during swallowing in adult males. *Br J Orthod*, **2**, 121–125.

Larsson, E. (1972) Dummy and finger sucking habits with special attention to their significance for facial growth and occlusion. 5. Improvement of malocclusion after termination of the habit. *Swed Dent J*, **65**, 635–642.

Larsson, E. (1988) Treatment of children with a prolonged dummy or finger-sucking habit. *Eur J Orthod*, **10**, 244–248.

Modeer, T., Odenrick, L. & Lindner, A. (1982) Sucking habits and their relation to posterior cross bite in 4 year old children. *Scand J Dent Res*, **90**, 323–328.

Moss, J. P. (1980) The soft tissue environment of teeth and jaws. An experimental and clinical study. Part 1. *Br J Orthod*, **7**, 127–137.

6

Dental factors affecting occlusal development

The size of the dentition in relation to jaw size

The third major factor affecting the development of the occlusion of the teeth is the relationship between the size of the dentition and the size of the jaws which have to accommodate the teeth. Ideally, there should be adequate space for the teeth to erupt into the mouth without crowding or overlap. It has already been shown that in the primary dentition the ideal situation exists when there is spacing between the anterior teeth, there being then a better chance that the permanent teeth will not be crowded. In the permanent dentition, contact between adjacent teeth is regarded as correct, though slight spacing is usually accepted as satisfactory. In present day mixed populations these ideals are realized all too seldom, particularly in the permanent dentition. In the primary dentition, actual overlapping of the teeth is unusual, and a disproportion between jaw size and tooth size is usually manifested as a lack of spacing rather than as actual crowding. Foster *et al.* (1969) found that the mean primary dentition size was very slightly less than the mean dental arch size in a population of $2\frac{1}{2}$-year-old British children, and Foster and Hamilton (1969) found only 1% of primary dentitions with no spaces in the dental arch in a similar population. These findings agree with those of other investigators, who have generally found that the mean dental arch length slightly exceeded the mean mesio-distal dimension of the primary dentition. In the permanent dentition, however, crowding of the teeth is much more common. Lavelle and Foster (1969) in a quantitative assessment of dentition and dental arch size in an adult British population, found that more than 65% of the population had a larger dentition than dental arch, and therefore had crowding of the teeth. Foster and Day (1974) in a clinical study of crowding in 11–12 year old British children found that 60% had actual or potential crowding of the permanent dentition (Fig. 6.1).

The aetiology of dental arch crowding has been the subject of several theories. It has been suggested that there is an evolutionary trend towards a diminution in size of the jaws without a corresponding diminution in tooth dimensions. This theory has received support from the studies of Moore *et al.* (1968) on the dimensions of jaws and teeth from Neolithic to modern times. It has also been suggested that dietary factors may be involved, the modern diet needing less chewing and

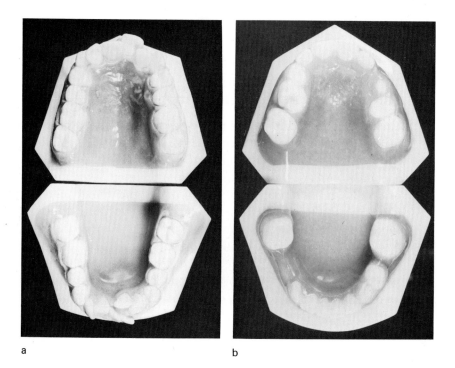

a   b

Fig. 6.1. (a) Actual crowding of the teeth. (b) Potential crowding—there is insufficient space for the remaining teeth to erupt into the arch.

therefore providing less stimulus to jaw growth than the more primitive diets. There is little evidence to support this theory. A further theory postulates that present-day populations represent a mixture of peoples from various ethnic backgrounds, and such interbreeding of people with different physical characteristics leads to skeletal and dental disharmonies. There is evidence for the independent genetic control of tooth size and jaw size, and this may in part explain the high prevalence of crowding of the teeth.

Dental arch crowding is not, however, only a feature of modern populations. Dickson (1969) has pointed out that it existed in primitive man and in pre-human species. Indeed, it has been so common that it is considered by some to be the normal state, rather than an abnormality. Fig 6.2 shows skulls from the 6th century AD which exhibit crowding and irregularity of teeth such as is frequently seen today. The question remains whether crowding of the teeth is more prevalent or more severe today than at previous times, and in the absence of previous epidemiological studies this question is difficult to answer. From the evidence

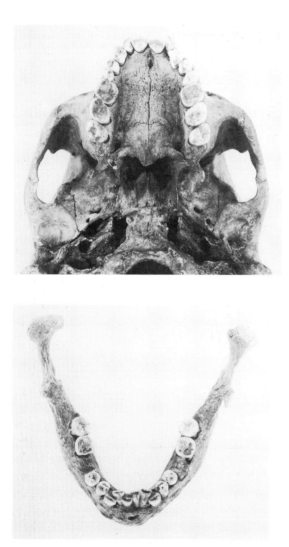

Fig. 6.2. Anglo Saxon jaws from the 6th century AD, showing crowding and irregularity of the teeth.

available it would seem likely that there is a higher prevalence of dental crowding in modern mixed populations than in many of the more pure ethnic groups, both past and present.

Thus, disproportion in size between the jaws and the teeth is a feature of many dentitions, but the main problems affecting occlusal development in this respect appear when the dentition is too large for

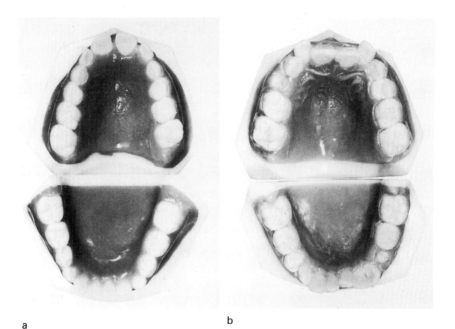

a   b

Fig. 6.3. The effect of dental arch size on crowding. Two subjects with similar-sized jaws and teeth. In (a) the dental arch has been spread and spaced by the muscles of lips and tongue. In (b) the dental arches have been constricted by lip activity and the teeth are crowded.

the jaws; a dentition too small for the jaws is only rarely a problem in orthodontic practice.

It must be remembered that disproportions in dentition size and jaw size do not always manifest as dental arch crowding. The form and size of the dental arch is important in governing the space available for the teeth, and, as has already been mentioned (see Chapters 4 and 5), the size of the dental arch may not be the same as the size of the arch of the basal bone of the jaw. Skeletal relationship and muscular factors can produce a dental arch which is larger or smaller than the arch of the basal bone, thus reducing or increasing the effects of excessive dentition size (Fig. 6.3). Therefore, in considering these effects, it is more realistic to consider dentition size in relation to dental arch size, rather than to jaw size.

The effects of excessive dentition size

Excessive dentition size in relation to dental arch size can have the following effects:

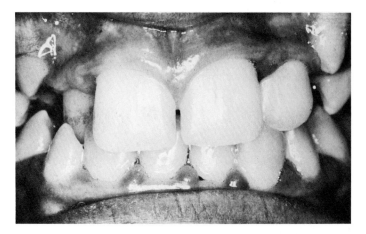

Fig. 6.4. Overlapping and displacement of teeth, causing problems with functional and artificial cleansing.

1 Overlapping and displacement of teeth.
2 Impaction of teeth.
3 Space closure after extractions.

OVERLAPPING AND DISPLACEMENT OF TEETH

When the dental arch is too small for the dentition, teeth erupting into the arch tend to become displaced by teeth already in the arch. This particularly affects the last teeth to erupt in any group, the lateral incisors, second premolars, canines and third molars. In the incisor region, the teeth tend to overlap, a condition often called imbrication, though imbrication strictly refers to overlapping like tiles, i.e. all in the same direction. In the buccal segments, the teeth tend to be displaced out of the arch (Fig. 6.4).

These conditions interfere with functional and artificial cleansing of the teeth, and usually warrant treatment if severe.

IMPACTION OF TEETH

Impaction of teeth occurs when eruption is completely blocked by other teeth due to crowding. Again, it tends to affect the last teeth to erupt in each segment (Fig. 6.5). The conditions in which teeth will become impacted rather than be diverted to erupt in aberrant positions are not understood, though the original position of the erupting tooth is probably important.

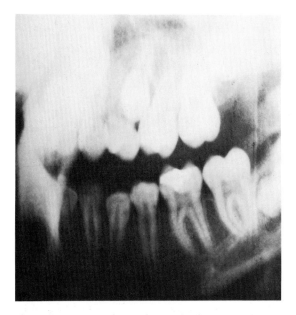

Fig. 6.5. Impaction of second premolar due to crowding.

SPACE CLOSURE AFTER EXTRACTIONS

There have been many investigation into spontaneous space closure after extraction of teeth. Seipel (1946) found that in the primary dentition space closure occurred less in the incisor region than in the molar region, and more in the upper arch than in the lower. He also found that in the primary dentition, space closure after extractions was progressive up to 28 months after the extractions, but in the permanent dentition space closure proceeded most rapidly for the first 3 months, slowed a little up to 9 months, and then slowed considerably, with little space closure thereafter. He found that the most important factor in governing the amount and rate of space closure was the degree of crowding of the dental arch, a finding that has been confirmed by most investigators (Inoue *et al.* 1983). Northway *et al.* (1984) also found that more space closure occurred in the upper arch than in the lower.

It is fairly generally accepted that space closure is dependent mainly on the relationship between dental arch size and dentition size. If the dentition is small in relation to the dental arch, little or no space closure will occur as a result of loss of teeth. The dental arch may be spaced, and the spaces would not be expected to close after full development of the occlusion. If, on the other hand, the dentition is large in relation to dental

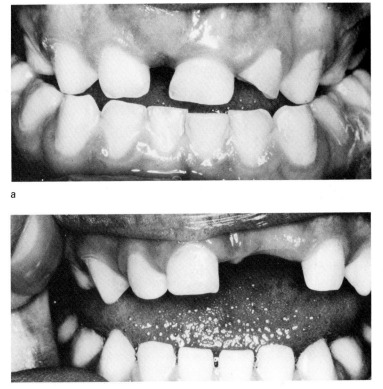

a

b

Fig. 6.6. Space closure in the primary incisors is dependent on the crowding potential. In both cases, an upper primary central incisor has been lost. In (a) no spacing in the lower primary incisors indicates potential crowding of the permanent teeth, and the extraction space has largely closed. In (b) a spaced lower primary arch indicates no crowding potential, and the extraction space has not closed.

arch size, tooth movement will occur to close any spaces unless some physical obstruction to such movement is present, e.g. interlocking cusps (Fig. 6.6).

It is also generally accepted that space closure after extractions in a crowded or potentially crowded dental arch occurs from both sides of the extraction space, i.e. both mesial movement of the teeth behind and distal movement of the teeth in front of the space. (Northway *et al.* 1984). Unless there is some physical barrier, the mesial movement usually exceeds the distal movement, perhaps by a factor of two to one.

Space closure is particularly important in relation to the premature loss of primary teeth, when teeth on each side of the residual space may move into the space. This can be considered with other effects of early loss of primary teeth.

The effects of early loss of primary teeth

The primary dentition has for long been the subject of difference of opinion regarding its value and the need for its preservation. It has been said that, as the primary dentition is of only temporary nature, its preservation is not important, and the premature loss of a primary tooth has usually been accepted more calmly than the loss of a permanent tooth. On the other hand, it has also been said that the presence of the primary dentition is essential for normal growth of the jaws, for normal function and eventually for normal position and occlusion of the permanent teeth, and that the premature loss of a primary tooth is to be avoided if at all possible.

To investigate the merits of these opposite viewpoints it is necessary to examine the effects which have been claimed following premature loss of primary teeth. These effects can be considered under the following headings:

1   Function and oral health.
2   Over-eruption of opposing teeth.
3   Psychological effects on child and parent.
4   Position of permanent teeth.

EFFECTS ON FUNCTION AND ORAL HEALTH

Early loss of primary teeth may affect masticatory function, but, with the modern diet, the effects are likely to be small unless most or all of the teeth are lost. Even in the latter case it is debatable whether the effects on masticatory function are sufficiently severe to cause digestive problems.

There may be slight effects on speech following loss of anterior primary teeth, but these are likely to be transient.

As far as oral health is concerned, the immediate effects of loss of infected primary teeth may be beneficial, removing stagnation areas and clearing oral sepsis. It has also been claimed that the loss of certain primary teeth, particularly the first molars, reduces the incidence of dental caries in the remaining teeth. There are, however, other methods of dealing with oral sepsis and of preventing dental caries without the loss of teeth, and the longer term effects of tooth loss also need to be considered.

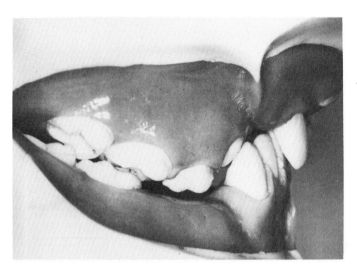

Fig. 6.7. Excessive vertical development of dento-alveolar structures following loss of primary teeth. This is usually a transient feature, the occlusal levels being adjusted as the permanent teeth erupt.

OVER-ERUPTION OF OPPOSING TEETH

When a tooth is lost from the dental arch, excessive eruption of the opposing tooth, or excessive vertical dento-alveolar development, frequently occurs. This can be seen following loss of primary teeth (Fig. 6.7), but on the whole this effect is transient. The eventual eruption of the successional teeth, together with continued alveolar growth, usually result in the establishment of the correct occlusal plane, provided the successional teeth meet in occlusion.

PSYCHOLOGICAL EFFECTS ON CHILD AND PARENT

Undoubtedly, the loss of anterior primary teeth alters the appearance of the child, which in some cases may produce undesirable psychological effects. After the age of 6 years most children and parents accept the natural loss of anterior primary teeth, but when these teeth are lost at an earlier age some parents, though not usually the children, are concerned by the appearance of the remaining dentition.

The other main psychological effect of losing primary teeth is that of 'losing the battle' against dental disease. The loss of a tooth is considered in this light by some parents and children, particularly if efforts have previously been made to save the tooth. The child's and the parent's attitudes towards dental health and dental care may be influenced by the attitude of the dentist towards preservation of the primary dentition. Any suggestion that the primary dentition is unimportant or that primary teeth are expendable may be reflected in an unfavourable attitude to dental care on the part of the child or parent. If primary teeth need to be removed it is better that they are lost as part of a plan for the benefit of the child, rather than as a result of a failure of dental care.

EFFECTS ON THE POSITION OF PERMANENT TEETH

As far as the occlusion and position of the teeth is concerned, the most important result of premature loss of primary teeth is space closure, but this does not mean that premature loss is necessarily a disadvantage to the ensuing occlusion. The movement of teeth which will occur in potentially crowded jaws may even prove advantageous, by localizing the crowding to one part of the dental arch instead of allowing it to be spread around the arch.

From a consideration of the factors involved in space closure, the following categories of conditions can be outlined, in which premature loss of primary teeth may have adverse effect or no adverse effect on the position of the permanent teeth.

(a) When there is ample space in the dental arch (Fig. 6.8a) to accommodate all the successional teeth, little or no space will be lost by spontaneous movement following loss of primary teeth, and no crowding of the permanent teeth is likely to ensue.

(b) When there is just enough space for the successional teeth to erupt without crowding (Fig. 6.8b) the loss of even a small amount of space by movement of teeth into an extraction space will result in crowding of the permanent teeth. Therefore consideration of the ensuing occlusion must be added to other considerations in planning the management of the primary dentition.

(c) When there is slight crowding potential in the dental arch for the successional teeth (Fig. 6.8c) it can only be relieved by the loss of permanent teeth. It is usually desirable in this circumstance to remove teeth symmetrically from each side of the arch. Therefore slight crowding of the permanent teeth in one arch would normally be corrected by the loss of two permanent teeth from that arch. This may result in the creation of more space than is necessary to relieve the

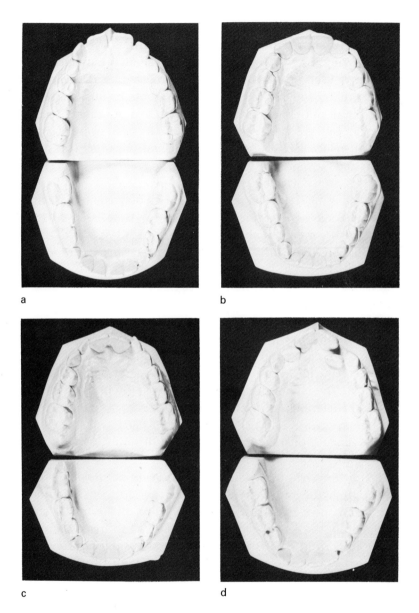

a
b
c
d

Fig. 6.8. Four conditions in which premature loss of primary teeth will have different effects on the occlusion. (a) Ample space in the arch. No space loss will occur. (b) Just enough space for successional teeth. The loss of primary teeth may result in some space loss and therefore avoidable crowding. (c) Slight crowding potential. Crowding of the arch is unavoidable, and loss of primary teeth may be beneficial in localizing this crowding. (d) Severe crowding potential. Loss of primary teeth may increase the severity of the crowding and aggravate the problem.

crowding. The premature loss of primary teeth in such conditions of slight crowding potential will result in partial space closure, and an increase in the crowding potential. However, the extraction of two permanent teeth from the arch would probably be sufficient to relieve the crowding, and it is likely that there would be no adverse effect on the position of the permanent teeth from loss of primary teeth in this situation. Indeed, there is often a beneficial effect, because crowding is frequently localized in the premolar region following loss of primary molars and movement of adjacent teeth, and in this position crowding is usually readily corrected.

It must be remembered that the above comments make no allowance for the need for space to correct dental arch discrepancies, and therefore do not apply in the presence of Class 2 or Class 3 dental arch relationships which need correction (see Chapters 17 and 18).

(d) When there is severe crowding potential in the dental arch for the successional teeth, (Fig. 6.8d) the eventual removal of a permanent tooth from each side of the dental arch may barely provide sufficient space for the remaining teeth. In such circumstances the premature loss of primary teeth can be expected to result in marked movement of teeth into the extraction space, with consequent aggravation of the crowding potential. The loss of primary teeth in these conditions will therefore have an adverse effect on the ensuing occlusion of the teeth.

The effects of asymmetric loss of primary teeth

In a crowded arch, if the loss of primary teeth occurs only on one side of the arch the resultant distal movement of teeth anterior to the extraction space can lead to an asymmetry of the dental arch, with deviation of the centre, which can be difficult to treat. Therefore, in a crowded arch it is best to plan for lateral symmetry of extraction of primary teeth if any primary teeth have to be lost (Avramaki & Stephens 1988).

The assessment of the potential space for the teeth

It is obvious that in order to apply the above considerations to the assessment of the effects of premature loss of primary teeth it is necessary to be able to assess the potential space available for the successional teeth. This involves assessment of both the space available in the dental arches and the size of the successional dentition. The first can be readily assessed by observation or direct measurement. The second is more difficult, since the teeth are unerupted. Measuring the space condition does not necessarily give an accurate assessment of space loss by spontaneous movement of teeth, but, relative arch crowding being the most important factor in space loss, such measurement is the most accurate method of prediction.

Two methods of assessment are commonly used, direct observation and mixed dentition analysis.

DIRECT OBSERVATION

Direct observation of the size of the dental arch or the space into which the successional teeth must fit is simple enough, but it must be coupled with an assessment of the size of those teeth, and this requires clinical experience. Some idea of permanent tooth size can be gained from the size of the primary teeth, though it has been mentioned previously that the correlation between primary dentition size and permanent dentition size is not strong (Lysell & Myrberg 1982). Radiographs of the unerupted teeth can give a better idea of their size in relation to the size of the dental arch, particularly if due allowance is made for magnification of the radiographic image.

Although it might be expected that jaw growth will increase the available space for the teeth, it is difficult to allow for the effects of growth because there is so much individual variation. Several observers have shown that the dental arch changes little, or actually decreases in size after the permanent dentition erupts. Generally speaking, therefore, it is probably better not to allow for jaw growth in the assessment of potential space for the teeth, and indeed it may be best to err on the side of pessimism, particularly as in potentially crowded dentitions spontaneous movement of teeth tends to reduce available space and negate the effects of jaw growth.

MIXED DENTITION ANALYSIS

A more accurate assessment of the potential spacing condition of the permanent successional teeth can be made by using some form of mixed dentition analysis. At its simplest, this involves measurement of the space available for permanent canines and premolars and radiographic measurement of the size of the unerupted teeth. Ingervall and Lennartsson (1978) have reported this to be the most accurate method of analysis.

A more sophisticated type of mixed dentition analysis is based on probability tables which give the widths of the permanent canines and premolars at various levels of probability, determined from the measured widths of the permanent incisor teeth. The procedure involved is first to measure the widths of the four permanent incisors in the appropriate jaw, and the distance between the second incisor and the first permanent molar, i.e. the space available for the successional canines and premolars. Then the probable widths of the successional teeth are determined from the probability table, at any desired level of probability, the conventional level being 75%. Finally, 1.7 mm is subtracted from the space available for the successional teeth in any one quadrant to allow for forward movement of the first permanent molar. It can then be seen whether the successional canines and premolars are likely to fit into the space available, and if not, an appropriate decision can be taken, using the rationale outlined above, as to whether the premature loss of a primary molar will have any adverse effect on the developing occlusion. Probability tables, have been produced by Staley *et al.* (1979) and by Bishara and Staley (1984).

This type of mixed dentition analysis probably gives a fairly accurate assessment although Lysell and Myrberg (1982) consider them to be of limited clinical value. Unfortunately, probability tables for dentition size are only available for a few localized populations, and to transfer probability tables from one population to another would reduce their accuracy.

Space maintenance

It will be realized from what has been said above, that, in some circumstances, the loss of one or more primary molars would have an adverse effect on the developing occlusion, by causing critical space loss. It is likely that these circumstances do not occur often, and when they do it may well be possible to preserve the primary teeth long enough to prevent space loss, but, if the primary teeth must be removed, some method of maintaining the space until the successional teeth erupt would be desirable. There has been a good deal of difference of opinion regarding the use of artificial space maintainers after early loss of primary teeth. While some clinicians employ them regularly, Inoue *et al.* (1983) have concluded, from a study of space closure after extraction, that space maintainers are not useful because they are not necessary in conditions of minor space deficiency and not effective when there is severe space discrepancy. There certainly does not seem to be any case

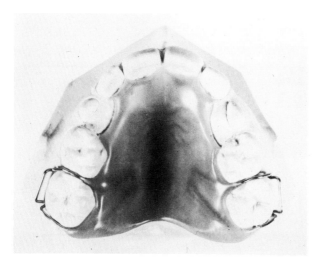

Fig. 6.9. Removable space maintainer to allow eruption of the permanent canines after removal of the first premolars.

for the routine use of artificial space maintenance, and even in those circumstances where space maintenance may benefit the developing occlusion other problems may arise from their use. If a space maintainer has to be worn for a long period there is some chance of damage to oral tissues through interference with cleansing, and this must be borne in mind when deciding whether to fit a space maintenance appliance after premature loss of a primary tooth.

There are many different types of space maintainer, and they fall into two main categories, removable and fixed. The removable space maintainer (Fig. 6.9) may be used for relatively short periods, say up to 1 year. The fixed space maintainer (Fig. 6.10), if properly designed, is rather less damaging to oral tissues than the removable space maintainer, and less of a nuisance to the patient. It may therefore be used for longer periods, say up to 2 years. If a space maintainer would be needed for longer than this time, serious consideration should be given to the effects on oral health, and to the alternative of allowing space to close and later correcting the ensuing malocclusion. It should be emphasized that, whenever a space maintainer is fitted, regular attention must be given to its possible damaging effects on oral health.

The importance of the primary dentition

The foregoing comments have been made in an attempt to rationalize an attitude towards the importance of the primary dentition. There is no

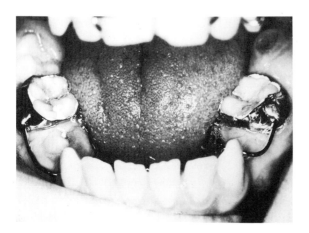

Fig. 6.10. Fixed space maintainers to allow eruption of the premolars after early loss of the primary molars.

doubt that if the primary dentition can be maintained in a healthy state, then, other things being equal, it should be so maintained for the benefit of the child. If circumstances make it difficult to maintain the primary teeth, such as severe dental disease or patient management problems, then in some cases primary teeth can be lost without adverse effects on occlusal development. In other cases the loss of primary teeth will be detrimental to occlusal development, and consideration will need to be given to preserving the teeth or fitting space maintainers. The other effects of loss of primary teeth, particularly the psychological effects on the child, will always need to be considered.

Summary

Crowding of the teeth is uncommon in the primary dentition. It is much more prevalent in the permanent dentition, where it can be found in over 60% of the British adult populations.

Aetiology of crowding—a disproportion between dentition size and dental arch size.

Dentition and dental arch size are probably under different genetic control. There may be some reduction in jaw size in modern populations.

Effects of crowding

1 Overlapping and displacement of teeth.
2 Impaction of teeth.

3   Movement of teeth into spaces created by attrition or extraction of teeth.

Effects of early loss of primary teeth

1   Little adverse effect on function. Variable effect on oral health.
2   Localized over-eruption of teeth is usually transient.
3   Variable psychological effects on child and parent.
4   The main effect is the movement of teeth into extraction spaces. Unilateral extraction of teeth in a crowded arch can lead to asymmetry of the arch through distal movement of teeth in front of the extraction site.

Spontaneous space closure

The most important predisposing factor is disproportion between dental arch and dentition size, i.e. crowding potential.

Conditions in which early loss of primary molars will give varying results

1   Ample space for the successional teeth. Little space loss is likely.
2   Just enough space for the successional teeth. Slight space loss will result in crowding potential.
3   Slight crowding potential. Space loss will aggravate crowding condition, but not beyond the scope of corrective treatment already necessary.
4   Severe crowding potential. Further space loss is undesirable.

Mixed dentition analysis

A method of assessing potential space condition of the successional teeth.

Space maintenance

Space maintenance by preservation of primary teeth or by removable or fixed space maintainers, should be considered if space loss is likely and is undesirable. Oral health problems may arise from the long-term use of artificial space maintainers.

References

Avramaki, E. & Stephens, C. D.(1988) The effect of balanced and unbalanced extraction of primary molars on the relationship of incisor centrelines—a pilot study. *J Paedr Dent,* **4**, 9–12.

Bishara, S. E. & Staley, R. N. (1984) Mixed dentition mandibular arch length analysis: a step-by-step approach using the revised Hixon–Oldfather prediction method. *Am J Orthod,* **86**, 130–135.

Dickson, G. C. (1969) The natural history of malocclusion. *Dent Practit,* **20**, 216–232.

Foster, T. D. & Day, A. J. W. (1974) A survey of malocclusion and the need for orthodentic treatment in a Shropshire school population. *B J Orthod,* **1**, 73–'78.

Foster, T. D. & Hamilton, M. C. (1969) Occlusion in the primary dentition. *Br Dent J,* **126**, 76–79.

Foster, T. D., Hamilton, M. C. & Lavelle, C. L. B. (1969) Dentition and dental arch dimensions in British children at the age of $2\frac{1}{2}$ to 3 years. *Arch Oral Biol,* **14**, 1031–1040.

Ingervall, B. & Lennartsson, B. (1978) Prediction of breadth of permanent canines and premolars in the mixed dentition. *Angle Orthod,* **48**, 62–69.

Inoue, N. (1983) Influence of tooth-to-denture-base discrepancy on space closure following premature loss of deciduous teeth. *Am J Orthod,* **83**, 428–434.

Lavelle, C. L. B. & Foster, T. D. (1969) Crowding and spacing of the teeth in an adult British population. *Dent Practit,* **19**, 239–242.

Lysell, L. & Myrberg, N. (1982) Mesiodistal tooth size in the deciduous and permanent dentitions. *Eur J Orthod,* **4**, 113–122.

Moore, W. J., Lavelle, C. L. B. & Spence, T. F. (1968) Changes in the size and shape of the mandible and lower dentition from neolithic to modern times in Britain. *J Anat,* **102**, 573 (Abstr.).

Northway, W. M., Wainright, R. L. & Demirjian, A. (1984) Effects of premature loss of deciduous molars. *Angle Orthod,* **54**, 295–329.

Seipel, C. M. (1946) Variation of tooth position. *Svensk Tandläk Tidskr,* **39**, Suppl.

Staley, R. N., Shelly, T. H. & Martin, J. F. (1979) Prediction of lower canine and premolar widths in the mixed dentition. *Am J Orthod,* **76**, 300–309.

7

Localized factors affecting the development of the occlusion

The more localized features which may modify the development of the position and occlusion of the teeth will now be considered. These features appear as modifying factors much less frequently than the general factors discussed in the previous chapters, and their effect is, of course, not so widespread, but they are superimposed on the general factors and may provide additional complications to occlusal development. Alternatively, a local abnormality may be the only modifying feature present in an individual, the effect of the general factors being entirely favourable to the development of ideal occlusion.

The features to be considered are:

1 Aberrant developmental position of individual teeth.
2 The presence of supernumerary teeth.
3 Developmental hypodontia.
4 The labial frenum.

A further localized feature, thumb or finger sucking has already been considered in Chapter 5.

It is also convenient at this stage to discuss the aetiology of *buccal crossbite* and the factors which govern *incisal overbite*.

Aberrant developmental position of individual teeth

The developmental position of any tooth, before it erupts into the mouth, may be such that it cannot erupt into its correct position in the dental arch. Although any tooth may develop in this way, certain teeth seem to be affected more than others. The teeth most commonly seen to be developing in an aberrant position are the upper canines, the lower third molars, the upper central incisors and the lower lateral incisors, all in the permanent dentition.

Aberrant developmental tooth position may be the result of trauma, or may be of unknown aetiology. Although crowding of the dentition is a common cause of tooth malposition, crowding is not considered here as a cause of aberrant developmental position.

Trauma affecting developmental position

The teeth most commonly seen to be developing incorrectly due to trauma are the upper central incisors. The typical history is that the child received a damaging blow to the upper incisor region of the primary dentition, usually at the age of 4–6 years. The primary upper central incisor may have been impacted upwards into the alveolar process. Sometimes no such history can be elicited, which suggests that even relatively minor damage, not remembered by the parent, may affect the developing permanent incisors, although Howard (1969) suggests that when there is no history of trauma, and particularly when there is little or no dilaceration, the tooth may be congenitally displaced rather than traumatized. At a later date the permanent incisor fails to erupt, and radiographic investigation reveals:

1 That the crown is malpositioned.
2 That the root is dilacerated (Fig. 7.1).

An explanation of the sequence of events is outlined in Fig. 7.2. The damage to the primary incisor has probably occurred at the precise time and in the precise direction for this tooth to be driven against the developing permanent incisor crown, causing the permanent tooth to be displaced so that its crown lies near the horizontal plane. The root then continues to develop vertically, with consequent dilaceration. These teeth will not normally erupt into the dental arch, mainly because of the shape of the root, though alignment is sometimes possible with appliance treatment (MacCauley 1969; Kolokithas & Karakasis 1979).

Aberrant developmental position of upper canine teeth

The permanent upper canine is probably the tooth which most commonly develops in the wrong position. The cause of this is unknown, though it has been suggested that, as this tooth begins to develop in a much higher position than the other upper teeth and therefore has a longer eruptive path, it has a greater chance of becoming malpositioned during the early stages of development.

Space deficiency in the dental arch, which may result in the deflection of the erupting canine tooth buccally or its impaction within the arch, does not seem to be a factor in causing the primary malposition of the tooth which is so often seen. Indeed, Jacoby (1983) reported that 82% of a large series of malpositioned upper canine teeth had adequate arch space.

The malpositioned upper canine is a frequent problem in orthodontic practice. As the patient commonly presents with the tooth unerupted, it is necessary first to locate the tooth and decide on its position, and then to decide on treatment. These two aspects will be considered separately.

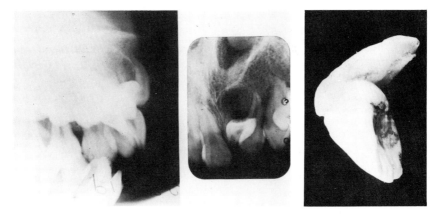

Fig. 7.1 Dilaceration and malposition of permanent upper central incisor as a result of early trauma.

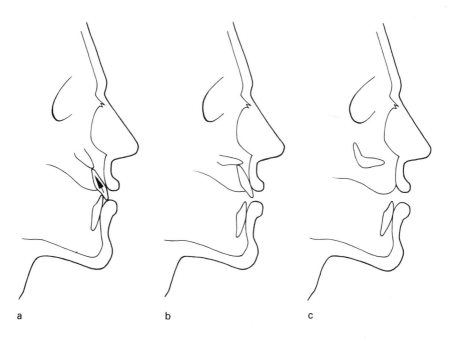

a   b   c

Fig. 7.2. (a) Trauma to the primary upper incisor may cause it to be impacted upwards against the developing permanent incisor. (b) The permanent incisor is driven upwards into a horizontal position. (c) The crown remains horizontal, but the root continues to develop vertically, resulting in dilaceration and failure of eruption.

Location of the unerupted malpositioned canine tooth

The assessment of the position of the unerupted canine involves visual examination, palpation and radiography.

VISUAL EXAMINATION

Apart from obvious swellings which may indicate the position of the crown of the tooth just below the surface of the oral mucoperiosteum, much can be gained by examining the upper lateral incisor. A developing canine tooth which is in or near the dental arch but inclined mesially may cause the root of the lateral incisor to tilt mesially and the crown to tilt distally (Fig. 7.3). Similarly, if the unerupted canine is positioned on the labial aspect of the alveolar process overlying the root of the lateral incisor, the lateral incisor root may be tilted palatally and the crown labially. An unerupted canine lying palatal to the dental arch does not usually cause any malposition of the lateral incisor, possibly because there is a greater depth of alveolar bone to accommodate the canine tooth in this region.

PALPATION

The palpation of the primary canine can sometimes give some indication of the position of the unerupted permanent canine. If the permanent canine is well away from its correct position it is unlikely to

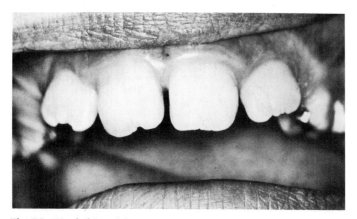

Fig. 7.3. Distal tilting of the permanent upper lateral incisors caused by mesial inclination of the upper canines.

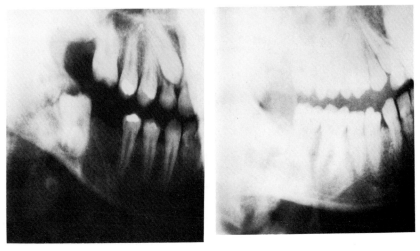

a   b

Fig. 7.4. Unerupted upper canines with mesial tilt, (a) resorbing, and (b) not resorbing the primary canine.

have caused resorption of the root of the primary canine, although the primary tooth may be resorbed at a later time. Therefore, if the primary canine is loose it is likely that the crown of the permanent canine is not far from its correct position, although the inclination of the tooth may be incorrect (Fig. 7.4). The permanent lateral incisor may have undergone resorption, and may be loose, though this is uncommon.

RADIOGRAPHY

The unerupted canine tooth can obviously be seen on a radiograph, but a single radiograph gives only limited information as to the position of the tooth. A two-dimensional film cannot give a true picture of the relative depth of the tooth. It is necessary to have at least two views of the tooth from different angles, and sometimes more views are necessary. The possible radiographic views are as follows.

1   Intra-oral (periapical)

This gives some indication of the inclination of the tooth, and of the degree of any resorption of the roots of the primary canine or permanent lateral incisor.

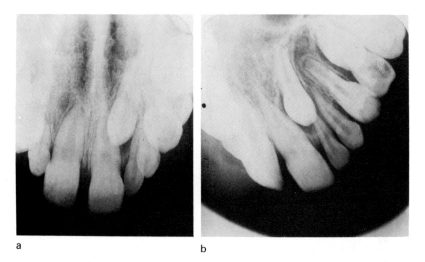

a   b

Fig. 7.5. Occlusal radiographs to assess the depth of an unerupted upper canine tooth.
(a) The straight anterior occlusal film shows the canine overlapping the central incisor.
(b) The oblique occlusal film shows the canine not overlapping the central incisor. For the
second film the X-ray tube has been moved distally and the canine appears to have moved
in the same direction, indicating from the principles of parallax that it is deeper than the
central incisor.

2   Anterior occlusal and oblique occlusal

These two views, observed in conjunction with each other, can, by
applying the principle of parallax, give an indication of the depth of the
tooth (Fig. 7.5).

3   Rotational tomograph

This view gives a good indication of the inclination of the unerupted
tooth (Fig. 7.6).

4   Postero-anterior and true lateral (extra-oral films)

These two views indicate the height of the tooth as well as the depth,
and to some extent the inclination. They suffer from the fact that several
other bony or dental structures may overlie the tooth in question,
making interpretation of the film more difficult.

The radiographic assessment of unerupted maxillary canines has
been well reviewed by Hunter (1981).

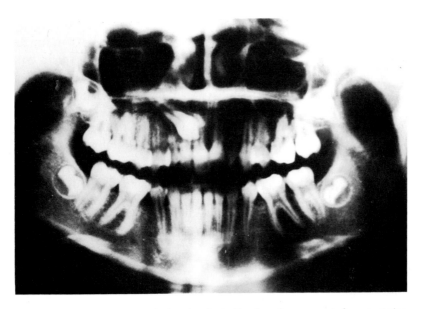

Fig. 7.6. Rotational tomograph showing the inclination of an unerupted upper canine tooth.

Treatment planning for the malpositioned unerupted upper canine tooth

Generally speaking, three treatment possibilities exist in this condition.
1   Removal of the tooth.
2   Alignment into the dental arch with appliances.
3   Immediate repositioning of the tooth, either by extraction and re-implantation or by immediate torsion.

Added to this is a fourth possibility of no treatment, i.e. the tooth is left unerupted. In such a case it would be necessary to maintain a regular review of the situation in case cyst formation or the resorption of other teeth occurred.

The following factors need to be taken into consideration in deciding on treatment.
1   The general state of oral health and the patient's age and desire to accept treatment.
2   The position of the unerupted tooth.
3   The space available in the dental arch.
4   The condition, position and appearance of neighbouring teeth, i.e. the lateral incisor, first premolar and primary canine.

5   The occlusal relationship of the dental arches.

As with much orthodontic treatment, the patient's willingness to maintain a good standard of oral health and to accept treatment is an important consideration. The alignment of an unerupted canine tooth may involve prolonged treatment with appliances, and should only be undertaken in favourable circumstances.

The position of the unerupted tooth, particularly the position of its apex, is often the overriding factor in deciding treatment. Most malpositioned upper canines are in palatal relationship to the dental arch. Provided sufficient space is available in the arch it is often possible to move the crown of the tooth into its correct position, but it is much more difficult to bring about movement of the apex of the root of the tooth. If the apex is far from its correct position, therefore, the possibility for alignment is limited.

There must obviously be sufficient space available for the tooth in the dental arch, either with or without planned extraction of other teeth. It is important to remember that the permanent canine tooth is usually appreciably larger than the primary canine, and if the primary canine has only just enough space there will not be space for the permanent tooth without further extraction or tooth movement. Existing crowding of other teeth must also be considered. The loss of an unerupted canine tooth may give enough space to relieve crowding of other teeth in the dental arch.

The condition of the neighbouring teeth, from the viewpoint of whether they will take the place of the canine tooth, must be considered. Sometimes the primary canine, if it has an adequate crown and root, or the first premolar, if it has moved forward into contact with the lateral incisor, will be satisfactory components of the dental arch in the permanent canine position (Fig. 7.7).

Finally, the occlusal relationship of the dental arches must be considered. If space is required in the arch to reduce a Class 2 occlusal relationship, a fairly common condition, it may be that such space can be gained, on one side of the arch at least, from the loss of an unerupted canine.

If it is decided that the unerupted tooth should be retained and aligned, two methods of treatment are available, as mentioned above. In the first, the eruption of the tooth is facilitated, usually by surgical exposure of the crown, removing bone from that aspect of the crown towards which movement is needed. An appliance is fitted to the teeth to apply force to the crown of the canine in order to move it into

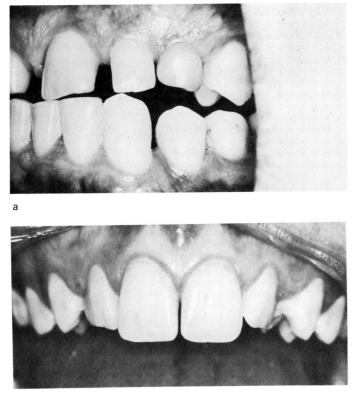

a

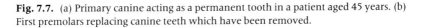

b

Fig. 7.7. (a) Primary canine acting as a permanent tooth in a patient aged 45 years. (b) First premolars replacing canine teeth which have been removed.

position in the dental arch. Several systems of appliance treatment can be used for this purpose.

The second method of treatment, immediate alignment, involves either the removal of the tooth and reimplantation into a socket prepared in the correct position in the bone, or immediate torsion of the tooth without removal, again into a prepared socket in the correct position.

In both cases the tooth must be held in position for a few weeks by means of a splint. Furthermore, reimplanted teeth must be clear of traumatic occlusal contacts. This type of treatment has been described by Sagne *et al.* (1986) and Kahnberg (1987), among others, and Northway and Konigsberg (1980) have given a comprehensive review of the ideal conditions and procedures for successful transplantation of teeth. The long-term results of replantation have yet to be fully evaluated, but there appears to be a reasonable measure of success over the first few years (Kahnberg 1987).

Breivik (1981) has shown that the odontoblasts of replanted immature teeth exhibit less degeneration and greater regenerative powers than those of mature teeth. This suggests that, if replantation is to be carried out, early treatment is likely to be more successful.

Aberrant developmental position of other teeth

As has been mentioned, any tooth can develop in the wrong position, though, with the exception of the lower third molars, such development of teeth other than upper canines is uncommon. The characteristic aberrant position of lower lateral incisors has been described by Taylor and Hamilton (1971) and is shown in Fig. 7.8. The deviations in developmental position of the lower third molar have been mentioned previously (see Chapter 3).

Supernumerary teeth

Supernumerary teeth occur more frequently in the premaxilla than in any other part of the jaws. They appear to be an inherited feature, no environmental factor having ever been shown to be responsible for their occurrence. The supernumerary teeth which appear so commonly in cleft lip and palate are probably the result of fragmentation of the dental lamina during cleft formation, and this cannot be considered as a normal circumstance.

There have been no reliable assessments of the prevalence of supernumerary teeth in various populations, though Stafne (1932) found supernumerary teeth occurring in about 1% of a large number of consecutive dental patients. They can occur in the primary or the permanent dentitions but only those in the permanent dentition have any marked effect on occlusal development.

Supernumerary teeth in the permanent dentition are of three main types.
1 Supplemental teeth—extra teeth of normal form.
2 Conical teeth—teeth with coniform crowns.
3 Tuberculate teeth—teeth with tuberculate or invaginated crowns.

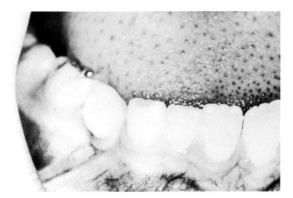

Fig. 7.8. Characteristic malposition of lower lateral incisor.

These types all have different characteristics and different effects on occlusal development.

Supplemental teeth

Supplemental teeth are supernumerary teeth of normal form. They appear most commonly, in Europeans, as extra upper lateral incisors and lower incisors in the permanent dentition, and may be present in the primary dentition (Fig. 7.9). It is less common to find supplemental premolars and molars, except in African and Asian populations.

The main effect of supplemental teeth on the occlusion is to increase the crowding potential. This does not always cause actual crowding, but frequently does so, particularly since crowding of the teeth is a common feature of modern populations.

It is often imposible to distinguish between the supplemental tooth and the normal tooth, and the supplemental tooth is not necessarily the one which needs to be removed to relieve crowding.

Conical teeth

The typical conical supernumerary tooth occurs in the premaxilla, near the mid-line, and is often called the *'mesiodens'* (Fig. 7.10). It may occur singly or in pairs, and occasionally more than two such teeth are present (Fig. 7.11). It is sometimes inverted, in which case it does not erupt into the mouth. Foster and Taylor (1969) have pointed out that the conical

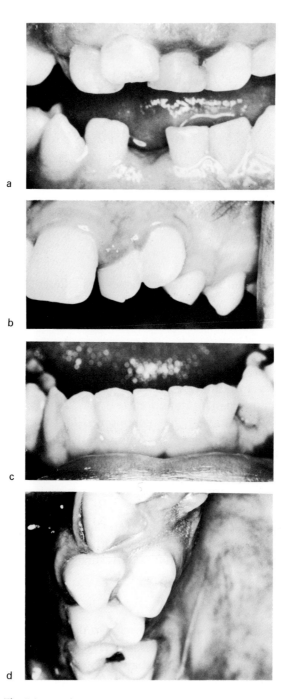

Fig. 7.9. Supplemental teeth. (a) In the primary dentition. (b) In the upper lateral incisor region. (c) In the lower incisor region. (d) In the upper premolar region.

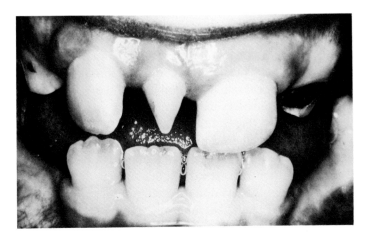

Fig. 7.10. The 'mesiodens'—a conical supernumerary tooth in the mid-line of the upper arch.

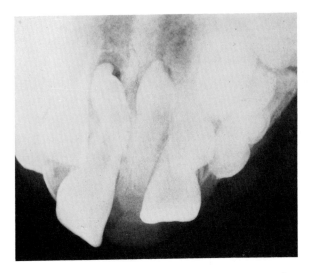

Fig. 7.11. Unerupted inverted conical supernumerary teeth.

supernumerary tooth has certain specific characteristics which distinguish it from the tuberculate tooth. The conical tooth appears to be an early development, its root formation being at least as early as that of the permanent upper central incisor, and sometimes earlier. It often erupts during childhood, and though it may cause malposition of the adjacent incisor teeth it does not delay their eruption to any great extent. Its most frequent position is between the permanent upper central incisors. Because of these characteristics it has been regarded as arising from the dental lamina as an extra tooth in the second dentition.

The occlusal problems caused by conical supernumerary teeth are usually confined to localized malalignment of the upper incisors. In particular, the central incisors may be rotated, or there may be a wide upper median diastema (Fig. 7.12). Treatment of these problems usually involves removal of the supernumerary tooth and local tooth alignment. Sometimes the supernumerary tooth is unerupted and causes no occlusal problems. In such cases the tooth may be left in place, particularly if it is high in the jaw and inverted, or if its removal would involve damage to other teeth. Any unerupted tooth not removed should be checked periodically, as mentioned earlier.

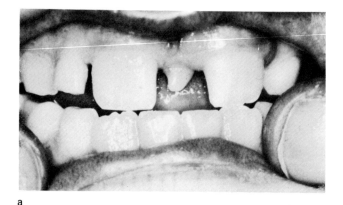

a

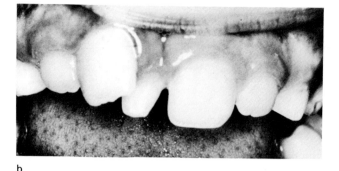

b

Fig. 7.12. (a) Upper median diastema and (b) displacement of upper central incisor associated with conical supernumerary teeth.

Tuberculate teeth

The tuberculate supernumerary tooth also occurs in the premaxilla, but is very different from the conical tooth, not only in form but also in position, behaviour, time of development and effect on other teeth. Foster and Taylor (1969) have shown that the tuberculate tooth is a later development than the conical tooth, its root formation being noticeably later than that of the permanent upper central incisor. It appears, characteristically, on the palatal aspect of the permanent central incisor, and does not normally erupt in childhood (Fig. 7.13). It may be unilateral or bilateral, and rarely is associated with supernumerary teeth of other types. Because of its late development and its typical position, the tuberculate tooth has been regarded as representing a third dentition.

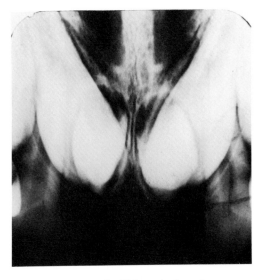

Fig. 7.13. Radiograph of bilateral tuberculate supernumerary teeth. The relative lack of root development compared with the development of the roots of the permanent upper central incisors can be seen.

The main effect of the tuberculate supernumerary tooth on occlusal development is that it delays the eruption of the permanent upper central incisor. Its presence is usually first suspected when the permanent lateral incisor erupts before the central incisor (Fig. 7.14). If the eruption of the central incisor is delayed, two problems may ensue. The lateral incisors may move medially, encroaching on the space which should be

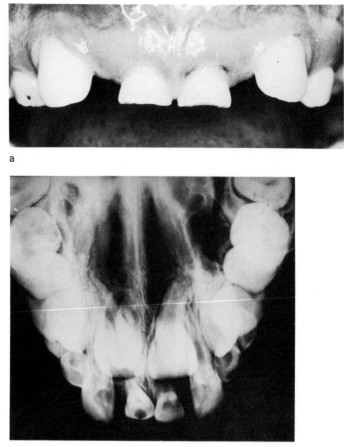

a

b

Fig. 7.14. The effect of tuberculate supernumerary teeth. (a) The eruption of the permanent upper central incisors is delayed, the primary central incisors being still present. (b) The radiograph shows the supernumerary teeth and the unerupted central incisors.

available for the central incisors. This is particularly likely to happen in conditions of potential arch crowding. Secondly, delay in eruption may cause reduction in dento-alveolar development in the vertical dimension, with the result that the central incisors, when they eventually erupt, remain on a higher level than the other teeth (Fig. 7.15).

It is therefore important that the tuberculate supernumerary tooth is removed as early as possible in order to prevent these developmental defects. If the tuberculate teeth are removed early enough, within a year

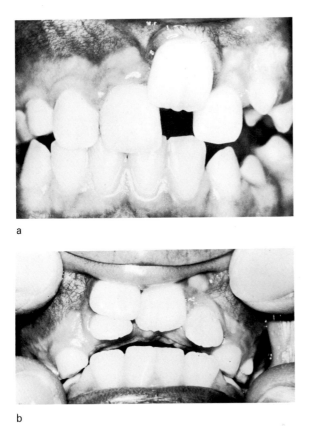

a

b

Fig. 7.15. The effect of delayed removal of tuberculate supernumerary teeth. Closure of the available space and failure of full eruption of the central incisor are common.

or so after the normal eruption time of the central incisors, the incisors will usually erupt into normal position (Fig. 7.16). Otherwise, orthodontic treatment to relieve crowding and move the lateral incisors distally and the central incisors vertically may be necessary after removal of the supernumerary teeth.

Developmental hypodontia

Hypodontia, the developmental absence of one or more teeth from the dentition, is not uncommon. Total anodontia is extremely rare, though cases are reported from time to time. Hypodontia, however, probably occurs in about 6% of European populations. Grahnen (1956) found

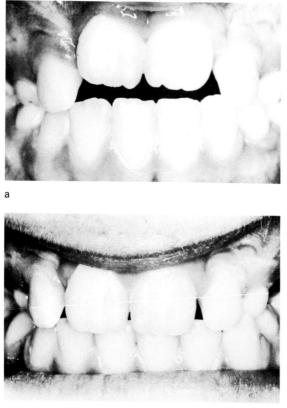

a

b

Fig. 7.16. Removal of tuberculate supernumerary teeth in good time will allow normal eruption of the central incisors.

6.1% of a population of Swedish children with one or more developmentally missing teeth, and Davies (1968) found hypodontia in 5.9% of a population of Australian children of European origin. These figures do not include the third molar, the developmental absence of which is difficult to assess with certainty in childhood. It seems likely that third molars are more frequently absent than other teeth.

Hypodontia appears to be an inherited characteristic. Although several other possible causes have been suggested, little evidence has been presented to support any cause other than genetic determination. It is common to find hypodontia as a family characteristic, though the precise genetic mechanisms responsible are not completely understood, and it is possible that there are several mechanisms of inheritance.

Hypodontia is sometimes associated with other forms of ectodermal dysplasia, such as sparse hair, a reduced number of sebaceous and sudoriferous glands and hypoplasia of finger or toe nails. A personal or family history of atopic dermatitis is often found. The condition has a wide range of severity, from the absence of one tooth to the absence of almost all the primary and permanent dentition, and the effects on the position and occlusion of the teeth and on jaw growth depend to a large extent on the number of teeth missing.

Certain teeth are missing more frequently than others. Grahnen (1956) found that in the permanent dentition the lower second premolar was most frequently missing (2.8%) followed by the upper lateral incisor (1.6%) and the upper second premolar (1.4%), and that of those with hypodontia, 85% had only one or two teeth missing. Similar proportions were found by Davies (1968).

The effect of hypodontia on dental occlusion

Hypodontia can modify the occlusion and position of the teeth by virtue of its effects on:
1 The form of the teeth.
2 The position of the teeth.
3 The growth of the jaws.

THE FORM OF THE TEETH

It seems that developmental hypodontia not only reduces the total number of teeth, but also may modify the shape of the teeth which are present. Foster and Van Roey (1970) have described the characteristic malformation of teeth which can occur in this condition. Incisors or canines may be coniform, cusp deficiencies may be seen on premolars and molars and various other malformations of teeth may occur (Fig. 7.17). Such malformation may be present even if only one tooth is missing, and indeed, occasionally a patient is seen who has no teeth missing, but who has malformation of teeth and a family history of hypodontia.

THE POSITION OF THE TEETH

Tooth position in hypodontia depends to a large extent on the number of teeth missing. Often, if only one or two teeth are absent, the effect is minimal, particularly when there would otherwise be a potential for

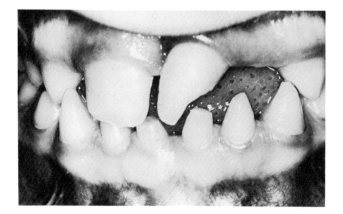

Fig. 7.17. Malformation of primary teeth and the permanent upper central incisor in severe hypodontia. No other permanent teeth were present.

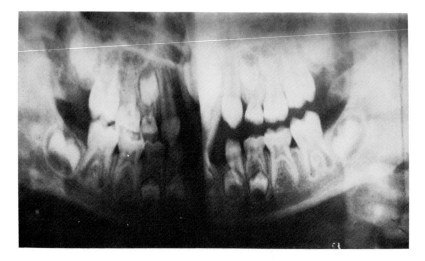

Fig. 7.18. Absence of second premolars. The primary molars may act as permanent teeth in such cases, if they are in good condition.

dental arch crowding. If several permanent teeth are missing, then, of course, there are likely to be spaces in the dentition, and teeth are likely to be malpositioned. This effect is sometimes alleviated by the presence of primary teeth, which may serve as permanent teeth in these circumstances (Fig. 7.18). If the primary teeth are also missing, then spaces may need to be closed by tooth movement, sometimes combined with the provision of dentures (Fig. 7.19).

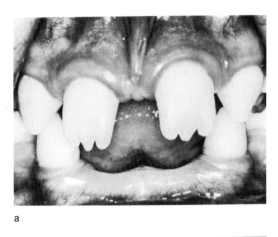

a

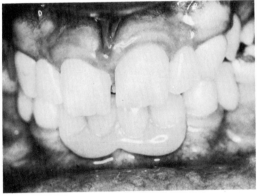

b

Fig. 7.19. (a) Hypodontia, with absence of upper lateral incisors and all the lower incisors. (b) Tooth movement and prostheses to replace the missing teeth.

THE GROWTH OF THE JAWS

Noticeable effects on jaw growth only occur in the more severe types of hypodontia, when a large number of permanent teeth are missing. The growth of the basal parts of the jaws is not affected, but the absence of much of the dentition causes reduction in growth of the alveolar bone. The vertical dimension of the face with the mandible in the rest position is unaffected, as this is dependent on muscular factors, but the vertical dimension in occlusion is reduced because of the reduced height of the alveolar process, and at rest there is an increased inter-occlusal clearance (Fig. 7.20). There is also reduction in transverse and antero-posterior dimension of the dento-alveolar structures, which is apparent

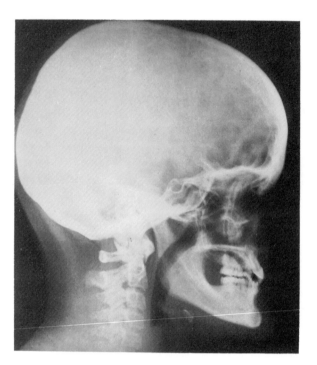

Fig. 7.20. Lateral radiograph of a child with severe congenital hypodontia. All the permanent dentition is missing except the upper central incisors. Note the small vertical dimension of the face when the teeth are in occlusion.

in the external facial appearance. Usually the provision of prostheses is necessary to replace the missing permanent teeth and to increase the dimensions of the jaws.

The upper labial frenum

The upper labial frenum occasionally causes localized modification to the position of the teeth. The labial frenum, in infancy, normally has a low attachment near to the crest of the upper alveolar process in the mid-line (Fig. 7.21). In the primary dentition the labial frenum can frequently be seen to be attached to the alveolar process between the upper central incisors. With normal dento-alveolar growth, the upper alveolar process grows down and the labial frenum attachment becomes progressively higher on the jaw. Occasionally, however, the low attachment persists, and the frenum apparently causes a mid-line space between the upper central incisors (Fig. 7.22).

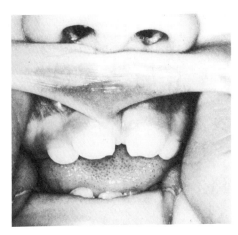

a

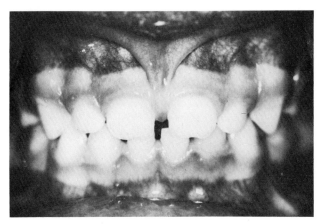

b

Fig. 7.21. (a) The normal attachment of the upper labial frenum in the infant at 10 months of age. (b) A low attachment of the labial frenum in the primary dentition at $2\frac{1}{2}$ years of age.

It is important to remember that there are other causes of upper median diastema, including the following:

1 Hypodontia, especially missing upper lateral incisors.
2 Proclination of incisors.
3 General spacing of the dentition.
4 The presence of unerupted conical supernumerary teeth.

Furthermore, a median diastema is often seen when the permanent incisors erupt, this being a normal feature in development, the diastema closing naturally as other permanent teeth erupt. A median diastema is

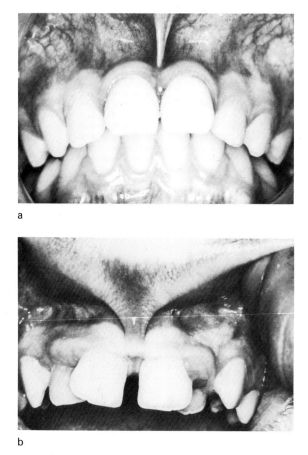

a

b

Fig. 7.22. (a) The normal attachment of the upper labial frenum in the permanent dentition. (b) A persistent low attachment of the labial frenum, associated with an upper median diastema.

also sometimes a familial characteristic, unassociated with a low frenum attachment or any of the features mentioned above.

Treatment to correct a median diastema caused by the low attachment of the labial frenum involves resection of the frenum, and appliance treatment to close the space between the teeth. Some spontaneous space closure can usually be expected after the frenum is resected, though the space will not usually close completely without appliance treatment. In view of the fact that several other factors may be responsible for the median diastema, it is necessary to be sure before carrying out frenectomy that the labial frenum is the main cause. A thick frenum, attached between the teeth, which causes blanching of the incisive papilla on being stretched, could reasonably be expected to be a prime cause of the median diastema, particularly if neighbouring teeth are crowded (Fig. 7.22). If there is doubt, it is probably best to wait until the permanent canines have erupted before carrying out frenectomy, to give maximum chance of spontaneous closure of the diastema during growth.

Buccal crossbite

Crossbite of the buccal teeth, i.e. when the teeth occlude with the buccal cusps of the lower teeth outside the arch of the upper teeth, may be bilateral or unilateral.

Bilateral crossbite

This is usually caused by the basal arch of the upper jaw being narrower than that of the lower jaw. It can also be the result of a positional discrepancy between the jaws, the lower jaw being too far forward in relation to the upper, the divergence of the mandibular arch towards the back producing a crossbite. It is commonly seen in subjects with Class 3 skeletal relationship, either because of a positional discrepancy or a size discrepancy between the jaws.

Bilateral crossbite is a symmetrical condition, and the mandibular path of closure from rest to occlusion usually occurs without lateral deviation.

Unilateral crossbite

This usually caused by the upper dental arch being slightly narrower than the lower dental arch. In this condition a central path of closure of the mandible would bring the buccal teeth into cusp-to-cusp occlusal contact, and there is usually a translocated path of closure into unilateral crossbite. Day and Foster (1971) have shown that unilateral crossbite is significantly associated with Class 3 Skeletal relationship, thumb sucking, adaptive swallowing behaviour and the presence of an instanding incisor. Presumably the first three of these features may cause slight narrowing of the upper dental arch, and the instanding incisor may cause initial contact and translocated closure into unilateral crossbite.

As *bilateral* crossbite is symmetrical, it is often considered to be acceptable. Orthodontic treatment to widen the upper dental arch sufficiently to overcome a bilateral crossbite is likely to relapse. It is possible to widen the upper jaw using rapid maxillary expansion techniques (Biedermann 1973) and it has been claimed that such techniques are valid since they widen the nasal airway and improve respiration (Hershey *et al.* 1976). However, Timms (1986), Hartergink *et al.* (1987) and Warren *et al.* (1987) have reported that these effects are of relatively minor degree and are not predictable. Since the success of rapid maxillary expansion depends largely on the widening of the mid-palatal suture and subsequent infilling with new bone deposition, it is not surprising that best results are claimed when used in patients who are still in the active growth phase (Bishara & Staley 1987). Linder-Aronson and Lindgren (1979) have reported that 5 years after treatment with rapid expansion the increase in intermolar width was 45% of the initial expansion, and there were no unfavourable side effects on the jaws or teeth, but Langford (1982) and Odenrick *et al.* (1982) have reported extensive root resorption resulting from rapid expansion technique.

Unilateral crossbite, when it involves deviation in the path of mandibular closure, usually warrants treatment. Its treatment by expansion of the maxillary dental arch is more realistic than in the case of bilateral crossbite, because much less expansion is needed. It is necessary, of course, to correct the aetiological factors as far as possible.

Buccal crossbite can occur in the primary dentition. Hanson *et al.* (1970) found crossbite in about 12% of a sample of primary dentitions, compared with about 16% in permanent dentitions (Foster & Day 1974). Thilander *et al.* (1984) and Schröder and Schröder (1984) have reported good results, from treatment of crosslite in the primary dentition phase.

The incisal overbite

The degree of incisal overbite shows a wide range of variation, from anterior open bite at the one extreme to complete overbite with the upper incisors more than covering the lower incisors at the other.

Overbite is determined by the degree of vertical dento-alveolar development in the incisor segment, and to some extent by the total height of the lower part of the face. At the extremes of the range of normal variation, an excessive facial height is likely to be associated with a high mandibular gonial angle and an anterior open bite, and a small facial height with a low gonial angle and a deep incisal overbite.

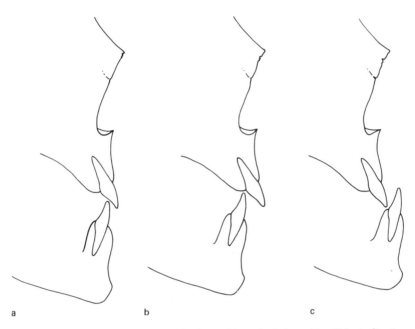

a   b   c

Fig. 7.23. The influence of the skeletal relationship on incisal overbite. If the inclination of the incisors remains constant, skeletal Class 2 (b) or Class 3 (c) discrepancy will allow excessive vertical development of the incisor segments, with consequent increase in overbite, provided no physical barrier intervenes.

Between these extremes, it seems unlikely that facial height and overbite are directly related, and overbite is governed more by the degree of dento-alveolar development in the anterior segments. These segments will usually continue to develop vertically until further growth is prevented by contact of the teeth on hard or soft tissue. An anterior open bite or an incomplete overbite is usually due to the tongue or the thumb preventing full vertical development.

If neither of these factors is present, then the degree of vertical development of the anterior segments will depend on the skeletal relationship of the jaws and the axial inclination of the incisor teeth (Figs. 7.23, 7.24). It can be seen that excessive incisal overbite will occur if the incisors are retroclined or proclined so that they fail to meet correctly, or if they fail to meet because of skeletal discrepancy. In all these circumstances vertical development may continue to an excessive degree.

In the Class 2 Division 1 occlusion vertical development of the lower anterior dento-alveolar segment is usually excessive, development of the upper anterior segment being limited by the lower lip. In Class 2

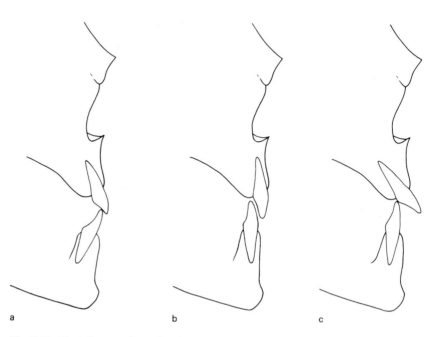

a   b   c

Fig. 7.24. The influence of incisal inclination on overbite. With the skeletal relationship constant, retroclination of the incisors (b) or proclination of the upper incisors (c) can result in increased overbite by allowing excessive vertical development of the anterior dento-alveolar segments.

Division 2 occlusion the lower lip usually functions in front of the upper teeth, and excessive vertical development of both upper and lower anterior segments can occur (Fig. 7.25). Treatment of excessive incisal overbite will be considered in Chapters 13 and 17.

Summary

Localized modifying factors may be superimposed on the general factors affecting occlusal development.

Aberrant developmental position of teeth

Developmental position may be affected by trauma, particularly of upper central incisors. Aberrant developmental position of unknown aetiology is most commonly seen in the permanent upper canines.

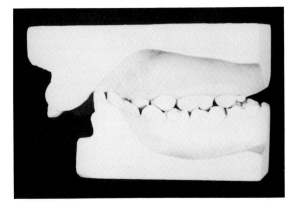

a

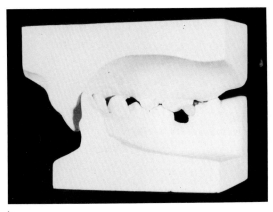

b

Fig. 7.25. Models of (a) Class 2 Division 1 occlusion; and (b) Class 2 Division 2 occlusion. Excessive vertical development has occurred in (a) the lower anterior segment; and in (b) the upper and lower anterior segments.

MANAGEMENT OF UNERUPTED UPPER CANINES

Location may be by means of visual examination, palpation or radiography.

Decision on treatment depends on oral health, patient co-operation, position of the tooth, space available, condition of neighbouring teeth and the occlusal relationship.

Treatment may be extraction, exposure and alignment, transplantation or immediate torsion.

Supernumerary teeth

There are three types of supernumerary teeth:

1 *Supplemental*—teeth of normal form.
2 *Conical*—usually near the mid-line of the premaxilla, the 'mesio-dens'.
3 *Tuberculate*—usually palatal to the upper central incisors, delaying their eruption.

Hypodontia

The developmental absence of teeth which occurs in about 6% of children. An inherited condition, sometimes associated with other forms of ectodermal dysplasia.

Effects on occlusion may be through:

1 The form of the teeth.
2 The position of the teeth.
3 The growth of the jaws.

The upper labial frenum

This may cause median diastema. Other possible causes are:

1 Hypodontia.
2 Supernumerary teeth.
3 General spacing of the dentition.
4 Proclination of the upper incisors.

Median diastema may be a normal phase of development, or a familial characteristic.

Buccal crossbite

Bilateral

Usually due to narrow upper basal bone, or Skeletal Class 3 relationship. A symmetrical feature, with central path of mandibular closure.

Unilateral

Usually associated with skeletal Class 3 relationship, thumb sucking, adaptive swallowing and instanding upper incisors. An asymmetrical feature, usually with lateral deviation in the path of mandibular closure.

Treatment is more desirable in unilateral crossbite, because of asymmetry and mandibular deviation.

Incisal overbite

This is governed by the degree of vertical growth of the anterior dento-alveolar segments, and at the extremes of the range of normal variation, may be related to lower facial height. Vertical development of the anterior segments usually continues until the teeth contact hard or soft tissue.

Anterior open bite and incomplete overbite are mainly caused by tongue activity or thumb sucking, rarely excessive lower facial height associated with high mandibular gonial angle.

Excessive overbite is usually due to antero-posterior skeletal discrepancy or proclination or retroclination of incisors, allowing excessive vertical development. Rarely, it is associated with small lower facial height and low mandibular gonial angle.

References

Biederman, W. (1973) Rapid correction of Class 3 malocclusion by mid palatal expansion. *Am J Orthod*, **63**, 47−55.

Bishara, S. E. & Staley, R. N. (1987) Maxillary expansion: clinical implications. *Am J Orthod*, **91**, 3−14.

Breivik, M. (1981) Human odontoblast response to tooth replantation. *Eur J Orthod*, **3**, 95−108.

Davies, P. L. (1968) Agenesis of teeth of the permanent dentition. A frequency study in Sydney school children. *Austr Dent J*, **13**, 146−150.

Day, A. J. W. & Foster, T. D. (1971) An investigation into the prevalence of molar crossbite and some associated aetiological conditions. *Dent Practit*, **21**, 402−410.

Foster, T. D. & Day, A. J. W. (1974) A survey of malocclusion and the need for orthodontic treatment in a Shropshire school population. *Br J Orthod*, **1**, 73−78.

Foster, T. D. & Taylor, G. S. (1969) Characteristics of supernumerary teeth in the upper central incisor region. *Dent Practit*, **20**, 8−12.

Foster, T. D. & Van Roey, O. (1970) The form of the dentition in partial anodontia. *Dent Practit*, **20**, 163−169.

Grahnen, H. (1956) Hypodontia in the permanent dentition. *Odont Revy*, **7**, Suppl 3.

Hanson, M. L., Barnard, L. W. & Case, J. L. (1970) Tongue thrust in pre-school children *Am J Orthod*, **57**, 15−22.

Hartergink, D. V., Vig, P. S. & Abbott, D. W. (1987) The effect of rapid maxillary expansion on nasal airway resistance. *Am J Orthod*, **92**, 381−389.

Hershey, H. G., Stewart, B. C. & Warren, D. W. (1976) Changes in nasal airway resistance associated with rapid maxillary expansion. *Am J Orthod*, **69**, 274−284.

Howard, R. D. (1969) The congenitally displaced maxillary incisor. *Dent Practit*, **20**, 361−370.

Hunter, S. B. (1981) The radiographic assessment of the unerupted maxillary canine. *Br Dent J*, **150**, 151−155.

Jacoby, H. (1983) The aetiology of canine impactions. *Am J Orthod*, **84**, 125–132.

Kahnberg, K. E. (1987) Autotransplantation of teeth; (1). Indications for transplantation with a follow up of 51 cases. *Int J Oral Maxillofacial Surg*, **16**, 577–585.

Kolokithas, G. & Karakasis, D. (1979) Orthodontic movement of dilacerated maxillary central incisor. *Am J Orthod*, **76**, 310–315.

Langford, S. R. (1982) Root resorption extremes resulting from clinical rapid maxillary expansion. *Am J Orthod*, **81**, 371–377.

Linder-Aronson, S. & Lindgren, J. (1979) The skeletal and dental affects of rapid maxillary expansion. *Br J Orthod*, **6**, 25–29.

MacCauley, F. J. (1969) Ectopic incisors. *Dent Practit*, **20**, 361–370.

Northway, W. M. & Konigsberg, S. (1980) Autogenic tooth transplantation. *Am J Orthod*, **77**, 146–162.

Odenrick, L., Lilja, E. & Lindbäck, K-F. (1982) Root surface resorption in two cases of rapid maxillary expansion. *Br J Orthod*, **9**, 37–40.

Sagne, S., Lennartsson, B. & Thilander, B. (1986) Transalveolar transplantation of maxillary canines. *Am J Orthod*, **90**, 149–157.

Schröder, U. & Schröder, I. (1984) Early treatment of unilateral posterior crossbite in children with bilaterally contracted maxillae. *Eur J Orthod*, **6**, 65–69.

Stafne, E. C. (1932) Supernumerary teeth. *Dent Cosmos*, **74**, 653–659.

Taylor, G. S. & Hamilton, M. C. (1971) Ecoptic eruption of lower lateral incisors. *J Dent Child*, **38**, 282–284.

Thilander, B., Wahlund, S. & Lennartsson, B. (1984) The effect of early interceptive treatment in children with posterior crossbite. *Eur J Orthod*, **6**, 25–34.

Timms, D. J. (1986) The effect of rapid maxillary expansion on nasal airway resistance. *Br J Orthod*, **13**, 221–228.

Warren, D. W., Hershey, H. G., Turvey, T. A., Hintory, V. A. & Hairfield, W. M. (1987) The nasal airway following maxillary expansion. *Am J Orthod*, **91**, 111–116.

8

The need for orthodontic treatment

Orthodontic treatment has a long history, the first recorded suggestions for active treatment being those of Aurelius Cornelius Celsus (25 BC–AD 50), who, in his seventh book on Medicine, advocated the use of finger pressure to align irregular teeth. Several other early writers advised the extraction of teeth to correct crowding and irregularity. In recent years the amount of orthodontic treatment provided has increased considerably, and several attempts have been made to define the need for orthodontic treatment.

The World Health Organisation (1962) includes malocclusion under the heading of Handicapping Dento-Facial Anomaly, which is defined as an anomaly which causes disfigurement or which impedes function, and which requires treatment *'if the disfigurement or functional defect is, or is likely to be, an obstacle to the patient's physical or emotional well being'*. Salzmann (1968) defines a handicapping malocclusion as one which adversely affects aesthetics, function or speech. Such general definitions are mainly of use in assessing the need for treatment in individual patients, and involve a large measure of subjective assessment.

Attempts have been made to assess occlusal conditions and the need for treatment objectively, usually for public health purposes. The former has proved to be more successful than the latter.

Assessment of occlusal features

Several indices of the occlusion have been made which, to a large extent, provide objective assessments (Van Kirk & Pennell 1959; Poulton & Aaronson 1961; Björk *et al.* 1964; Summers 1971). These indices have been devised by breaking down the occlusion into its more important component parts, such as crowding, spacing, antero-posterior relationship, incisal overjet and overbite, individual tooth malposition, etc., and assessing each component separately, using carefully defined criteria, or, where possible, actual measurement. The degree of deviation from the ideal for each component is scored, and the total score gives a measure of the degree of malocclusion. As the result of the assessment is a numerical score, it is more useful for public health purposes than for clinical purposes, where descriptive assessments are of **179** more value.

Assessment of need for treatment

Methods have been devised by Draker (1960), Grainger (1967), Salzmann (1968), Freer and Adkins (1968) and Freer (1972), among others, which have gone some way towards achieving objectivity in the assessment of treatment need for public health purposes (Gray & Demirgian 1977). Brook and Shaw (1989) have outlined a two-part index of orthodontic treatment piority. The first part assesses and scores factors of the occlusion and of oral health impairment, and the second part scores the degree of aesthetic impairment provided by malposition of the anterior teeth.

On the whole these methods involve the transfer of the results of assessments of occlusal features to an index of the need for treatment, on the basis that the higher the score for occlusal discrepancy the greater is the need for treatment. Therefore, although the occlusal assessment may be objective, such methods of assessing treatment need are based on the essentially subjective concept that certain deviations from the ideal occlusion would benefit from orthodontic treatment. Ideal occlusion is rare, and the degree of deviation from the ideal at which the need for correction begins has not been defined, and indeed may be impossible to define. An element of subjectivity in assessments of treatment need is therefore likely to remain.

Clinical assessment of treatment need

The reasons usually given for applying orthodontic treatment are the need for improvement in oral health, oral function and personal appearance. There is some evidence that malocclusion and malposition of the teeth can have an adverse effect on oral health, particularly on the condition of the periodontal tissues. Several studies have reported a significant relationship between irregularity of the teeth and dental plaque accumulation and periodontal disease (Behlfelt et al. 1981; Buckley 1981; El Mangoury et al. 1987; Addy et al. 1988). Clinical experience suggests that many aspects of malocclusion, e.g. excessive incisal overbite or severe irregularity of teeth, may affect oral health, and oral function may be adversely affected by such features as premature tooth contacts. On these grounds it seems reasonable to apply corrective treatment when it is felt that oral function and oral health will be improved, though there is little evidence that all orthodontic treatment provides such improvement.

Personal appearance does not lend itself to objective assessment, and the need for improvement depends to a large extent on the patient's or parent's wishes. There has, however, been an increasing interest in the alteration of the facial profile through orthodontic treatment. Attention has been paid to deviation from the ideals of facial form, and the possibilities for modification towards these ideals. Again, the question of need for change must inevitably be subjective.

The various methods mentioned above, which have been devised for assessing the need for treatment, are mainly for the assessment of populations, rather than for individual patients at a clinical level. For the individual patient, the following criteria may provide a realistic basis for the need for orthodontic treatment (see Chapter 2).

1 When there is a need for the subject to take up an adaptive postural position of the mandible.

2 When there is translocated closure of the mandible from the rest position or from an adaptive postural position to the intercuspal position.

3 When the tooth positions are such that adverse reflex avoiding mechanisms are set up during occlusal function of the mandible.

4 When the teeth are causing damage to the oral soft tissues.

5 When there is crowding or irregularity of the teeth which may predispose to periodontal or dental disease.

6 When there is adverse personal appearance caused by tooth position.

7 When the position of the teeth interferes with normal speech.

In such circumstances, if the movement of teeth and/or the planned extraction of teeth could achieve an improvement of the situation, then orthodontic treatment is necessary.

The application of these criteria will still involve a measure of subjective assessment, and even when the conditions listed above exist, it may not be possible to correct them by means of orthodontic treatment. Some of the more severe occlusal discrepancies are beyond correction in the present state of knowledge.

It seems likely that occlusal features and the level of need for orthodontic treatment vary between different population groups. The demand for orthodontic treatment also varies between different areas, being dependent not only on the need for treatment but also on socio-economic factors and on the availability of treatment services.

References

Addy, M., Griffiths, G. S., Dummer, P. M. H., Kingdon, A., Hicks, R., Hunter, M. L., Newcombe, R. G. & Shaw, W. C. (1988) The association between tooth irregularity and plaque accumulation, gingivitis and caries in 11–12 year old children. *Eur J Orthod*, **10**, 76–83.

Behlfelt, K., Ericsson, L., Jacobson. L. & Linder-Aronson, S. (1981) The occurance of plaque and gingivitis and its relationship to tooth alignment within the dental arches. *J Clin Periodontol*, **8**, 329–337.

Björk, A., Krebs, A. & Solow, B. (1964) A method for epidemiological registration of malocclusion. *Acta Odontal Scand*, **22**, 27–41.

Brook, P. H. & Shaw, W. C. (1989) The development of an index of orthodontic treatment priority. *Eur J Orthodont* **11**, 309–320.

Buckley, L. A. (1981) The relationship between malocclusion, gingival inflammation, plaque and calculus. *J Periodontol*, **52**, 35–40.

Draker, H. L. (1960) Handicapping labio-lingual conditions: a proposed index for public health purposes. *Am J Orthod*, **46**, 295–305.

El-Mangoury, N. H., Gaafar, S. M. & Mostafa, Y. A. (1987) Mandibular anterior crowding and periodontal disease. *Angle Orthod*, **57**, 33–38.

Freer, T. J. (1972) Assessment of occlusal status: the matched-pair similarity technic. *Int Dent J*, **22**, 412–422.

Freer, T. J. & Adkins, B. L. (1968) New approach to malocclusion and indices. *J Dent Res*, **47**, 1111–1117.

Grainger, R. M. (1967) *Orthodontic Treatment Priority Index*. Public Health Service Publication No. 1000, Series 2, No. 25. Washington DC, United States Government.

Gray, A. S. & Demirgian, A. (1977) Indexing occlusions for dental public health programmes. *Am J Orthod*, **72**, 191–197.

Poulton, D. R. & Aaronson, S. A. (1961) The relationship between occlusion and periodontal status. *Am J Orthod*, **47**, 690–699.

Salzmann, J. A. (1968) Handicapping malocclusion: assessment to establish treatment priority index. *Am J Orthod*, **54**, 749–765.

Summers, C. J. (1971) The occlusal index: a system for identifying and scoring occlusal disorders. *Am J Orthod*, **57**, 552–567.

Van Kirk, L. E. & Pennell, E. H. (1959) Assessment of malocclusion in population groups. *Am J Public Health*, **49**, 1157–1163.

World Health Organisation (1962) *Standardisation of Reporting of Dental Diseases and Conditions. 6. The Assessment of Handicapping Dentofacial Anomalies*. Technical report series, No. 242. Geneva, WHO.

9

Orthodontic tooth movement

Orthodontic treatment is based on the fact that it is possible, by applying appropriate forces, to move the teeth through the alveolar bone of the jaws without causing permanent damage to either the teeth or their attachment to the bone. It has long been known that such movement can be induced, but only in fairly recent times has experimental work been carried out in attempts to determine how the teeth move, the tissue reactions to forces applied to the teeth and the order of force necessary for satisfactory tooth movement. Even now, the detailed biological mechanisms of tooth movement are far from being completely understood, and many of the basic concepts are modified from time to time in the light of further research. In view of this, it is proposed to review some of the main investigations leading to the development of theories of tooth movement, and then to outline some more recent research which adds new interpretations to the older classical theories.

Investigations on tooth movement

When a force is applied to the crown of a tooth, it is transmitted through the root of the tooth to the periodontal ligament and alveolar bone. According to the direction of the force, there will be areas of pressure and areas of tension on these supporting structures. For the tooth to move, there must be resorption of alveolar bone in response to this stress, and if the tooth is to remain firmly attached there must also be deposition of bone to maintain the integrity of the attachment mechanism. In effect, the socket of the tooth must move, concomitant with movement of the tooth through the alveolar bone.

Although there had been previous observations and theories, Sandstedt (1904, 1905) was probably the first to investigate the phenomenon of tooth movement by histological examination of the supporting structures. Using orthodontic appliances on dogs, Sandstedt found the following:

1 Under gentle continuous forces, bone was resorbed from the 'pressure' side of the tooth socket, and new bone added to the 'tension' side, the newly formed bone spicules following the direction of the strained periodontal ligament fibres. There was no resorption of the tooth surface (Fig. 9.1a).

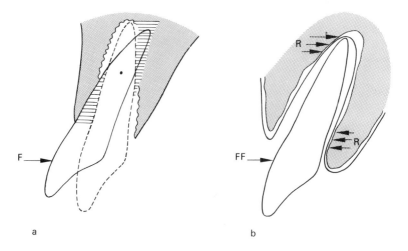

Fig. 9.1. Sandstedt's experimental findings. (a) Force on the tooth (F) causes tilting about a point near the centre of the root, and resultant resorption and deposition of bone from the periodontal ligament side of the socket wall. (b) Excessive force on the tooth (FF) produces areas of ischaemia in the periodontal ligament at the pressure sites, and subsequent undermining resorption of the socket wall from the endosteal side (R).

2 Under strong continuous forces, the periodontal ligament tissue was excessively compressed on the 'pressure' side, and no bone resorption occurred from the inner wall of the tooth socket. Within a short time, endosteal resorption of the socket wall occurred, a process referred to as *'undermining resorption'* by Sandstedt. Eventually the tooth moved as a result of this undermining resorption (Fig. 9.1b).

3 From the pattern of resorption and deposition of bone, it was concluded that the tooth tilted about a point near the centre of the long axis of the root.

Oppenheim (1911) experimented with orthodontic appliances on baboons, and later on dogs. His main conclusions were as follows:

1 In response to the force on the tooth, the alveolar bone on both pressure and tension sides was first transformed into a transitional osteoid tissue, laid down in the direction of the force, perpendicular to the surface of the root.

2 The transitional osteoid tissue was then resorbed on the 'pressure' side and new bone added on the 'tension' side of the socket.

3 The tooth tilted about a fulcrum near the root apex (Fig. 9.2).

Schwarz (1932) considered that Oppenheim's findings were histologically the same as those of Sandstedt, but that they had been interpreted differently. Schwarz went on to carry out his own experiments,

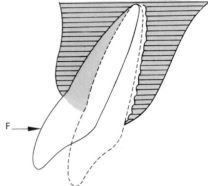

Fig. 9.2. Oppenheim's experimental findings. Force (F) applied to the tooth causes the whole of the supporting bone to be changed to a transitional osteoid tissue. Resorption of this tissue then occurs on the 'pressure' side, and deposition on the 'tension' side. The tooth tilts about the apex.

applying a range of forces to the teeth of dogs. He concluded that the most favourable tooth movement was produced by forces not greater than capillary blood pressure, such forces being insufficient to collapse the capillaries in the periodontal ligament. Schwarz outlined four degrees of biologic effect of varying forces on the teeth.

1   A force which is very slight, or of very short duration, causes no reaction in the periodontium.

2   A gentle continuous force, producing pressure in the periodontal ligament less than the pressure in the blood capillaries, results in resorption of alveolar bone at the regions of pressure, but no resorption of the tooth. Anatomical and functional normality returns after the force ceases.

3   A fairly strong force, which compresses the blood capillaries in the regions of pressure, results in ischaemia of the periodontal ligament. The resultant necrotic tissue becomes resorbed, and tooth resorption may occur. Functional normality of the periodontium, alveolar bone and root surface returns after the force ceases.

4   A strong force which crushes the periodontal ligament on the side of pressure, possibly causing contact between the tooth and the bone, results in undermining resorption from the endosteal surface of the socket. Tooth surfaces may also be resorbed. After the force ceases the tissues may return to functional normality, but there may be pulp death and possibly ankylosis between the tooth and the alveolar bone.

From his consideration of capillary blood pressure, Schwarz concluded that the optimum force for tooth movement was one which induced a pressure of $15-20$ g/cm^2 of root surface.

Reitan (1951) carried out a series of experiments on dogs and human subjects to determine the tissue reaction during tooth movement. Among his main findings were the following.

1 A transient dilatation of the capillaries in the periodontal ligament often followed the application of force to the tooth.

2 There was an increase in the cellular elements of the periodontal ligament, these being young connective tissue cells which had the potential for differentiation into formative or resorptive cells, i.e. osteoblasts or osteoclasts.

3 Bone resorption occurred on the 'pressure' side and osteoid tissue was formed on the 'tension' side. The osteoid tissue was more resistant to resorption than normal alveolar bone.

4 In circumscribed areas under heavier forces, 'hyalinization' of periodontal ligament tissue occurred, with reduction in the cellular element.

5 Under heavy forces, undermining resorption of alveolar bone occurred in circumscribed areas.

6 Tissue reactions occurred more rapidly in younger than in older subjects.

Many of the main conclusions of these investigators have been confirmed by other workers, and some modifications and further findings have been reported. Buck and Church (1972), experimenting on human subjects, found that even light tipping forces on the teeth resulted in extreme compression of the periodontal ligament with ischaemia and loss of cellular elements, probably through cell death. They did not consider that the resultant cell free areas could be considered as true hyalinization, as previously reported. They found that all resorption in the early stages was endosteal undermining resorption, and that when this resorption broke through to the periodontal ligament, cellular elements returned to the ligament. Storey (1973) has also suggested that repeated undermining resorption occurs, even with light forces. Khouw and Goldberger (1970), experimenting on monkeys and dogs, again found that force on the teeth resulted in occlusion of the periodontal ligament vessels on the 'pressure' side, but increased vascularity on the 'tension' side through distension of the blood vessels. However, after 7 days the vascularity was re-established on the 'pressure' side, and bone resorption progressed, with undermining resorption in some areas. On the other hand Rygh *et al.* (1986) found similar reactions to force on both the pressure and the tension sides, with intense vascular activity and the occurrence of macrophages in the periodontal ligament and in the alveolar bone.

Thus the tissue reactions to force on the teeth have been well documented, and although there is difference of opinion regarding some details, it would seem that the following reactions may occur as a response to force from orthodontic appliances.

1   Force not sufficient to occlude the blood vessels of the periodontal ligament

1   Hyperaemia within the periodontal ligament. Vessels dilate, though they do not necessarily increase in number.
2   Osteoclasts and osteoblasts appear in the periodontal ligament.
3   Resorption of bone of the lamina dura occurs from the periodontal side beneath the areas of pressure, accompanied by osteoclastic activity.
4   Apposition of osteoid tissue occurs on the inner surface of the socket beneath the areas of tension, accompanied by osteoblastic activity. This tissue becomes calcified within about 10 days, to form mature bone.
5   As the tooth and socket move through the alveolar bone, remodelling occurs to re-establish and maintain the integrity of the socket wall. This involves the addition of bone to the endosteal surface beneath the areas of pressure, and the resorption of bone from the endosteal surface beneath the areas of tension.
6   The periodontal ligament fibres attaching the tooth to the bone become re-organized. Progressive re-attachment occurs, possibly by the production of new fibres and attachment to existing intermediate fibres and to bone fibres which become progressively uncovered. The fibres which attach the tooth to the gingival tissue appear not to become re-organized, but are distorted as the tooth moves and may remain distorted for a considerable time.

2   Force sufficient to occlude the blood vessels of the periodontal ligament

1   Occlusion of blood vessels in the areas of pressure. Dilation of vessels in the areas of tension.
2   Appearance of cell-free areas in the periodontal ligament in areas of pressure.
3   Period of stasis, when the tooth does not move because no resorption occurs on the periosteal surface of the socket.
4   Increased endosteal vascularity, and endosteal resorption of the socket wall under the cell-free areas, i.e. 'undermining resorption'.
5   Relatively rapid movement of the tooth, accompanied by bone deposition within the socket beneath the areas of tension. The tooth may become slightly loose.
6   Healing of the periodontal ligament, re-organization of fibres and remodelling of the socket wall when forces are removed.

3 Grossly excessive force

If the force applied is severely excessive and prolonged the periodontal ligament in the areas of pressure will be deprived of its blood supply and there may be necrosis of the ligament, with massive undermining resorption and possibly resorption of the root surface of the tooth. This order of force is likely to be accompanied by pain, the tooth will become very loose and healing may be by ankylosis of the tooth to the alveolar bone.

Intermittent forces

The foregoing sequences of events occur when forces are continuous and steady. Intermittent forces in a constant direction have similar effects, though tooth movement may be slower, depending on the length of the intervals of rest between periods of force. Intermittent forces in alternately opposite directions can result in resorption of the apices of the teeth. Such forces usually occur when orthodontic appliances are worn intermittently, and, in the intervals, natural forces from the oral musculature act on the teeth in a direction opposite to that of the appliance.

The nature of tooth movement

Although the general nature of the cellular reactions to force on the teeth, which result in bone resorption and deposition, are not in dispute, the intermediary causes of these reactions have been the subject of more recent investigation. The classical theory of tooth movement suggests that the cellular reactions are simply the result of differential pressures induced in the periodontal ligament, and that the response to force is confined to the cellular elements of the ligament and the endosteal marrow spaces. This concept has been challenged by several investigators.

Baumrind (1969) has suggested that the ligament should be considered as a continuous hydrostatic system, in which differential pressures cannot exist. If this is so, the pressure–tension concept of the classical theory must be questioned.

The effects of *physical distortion of the alveolar bone* by the forces from orthodontic appliances may be responsible for the cellular reactions observed. Picton (1965), Cochran *et al.* (1967), Baumrind (1969) and Grimm (1972), among others, have shown that even relatively light forces on the teeth, such as are used in orthodontic treatment, cause bending of the alveolar bone. It has also been shown that bone which is deformed by stress becomes electrically charged, concave surfaces taking a negative polarity and convex surfaces a positive polarity (Epker & Frost 1965; Zengo et al. 1973). As a result of these bioelectric potential differences, bone is added to the concave surfaces and resorbed from the convex surfaces. In the dento-alveolar complex this would result in tooth movement (Tanne et al. 1987).

Justus and Luft (1970) have put forward a mechano-chemical hypothesis for the remodelling of bone under stress. Their experiments have suggested that altered physical stress in the bone changes the solubility of the hydroxyapatite crystals, which in turn induces the osteoblastic and osteoclastic activity which results in bone remodelling. Davidovitch et al. (1972) have also shown a biochemical process resulting from mechanically stressed alveolar bone to be an intermediate stage in bone resorption and tooth movement.

More recently the role of prostaglandins as mediators of tooth movement has been investigated. Prostaglandins are considered to be modulators of bone resorption and formation, locally produced as a result of physical stress (Sandy & Harris 1984). Yamasuki et al. (1984) have reported that the injection of prostaglandin E_1 to the alveolar bone in human subjects resulted in an almost doubled rate of tooth movement.

Gianelli (1969) confirmed, from experimental work, the previous findings of several investigators that an intact vascular perfusion system in the periodontal ligament seems to be necessary for frontal resorption of the bone, and that when the vessels are occluded by the force, undermining resorption occurs. He put forward the suggestion that the vasculature may act as a hydraulic pressure system, transmitting the applied force to the attachment apparatus, the resultant pressures distorting the crystal structure of the bone.

Mostafa et al. (1983) have postulated that force applied to a tooth produces two main effects, the periodontal tissue injury causing vascular responses and the bending of the alveolar bone causing piezoelectric responses and the local production of prostaglandins, all of which mediate tooth movement.

Thus there seems to be some evidence that the cellular reactions to force may be mediated by factors outside the periodontal ligament. The piezoelectric or mechanochemical effects of stress on the alveolar bone may be important factors in producing the osteoclastic and osteoblastic activity which results in tooth movement.

The forces involved in tooth movement

Although there is still doubt over the exact mechanisms of tooth movement, it is obvious that successful movement takes place with appropriate forces. According to Schwarz (1932), the ideal force is one which induces a pressure in the periodontal ligament not exceeding capillary blood pressure, i.e. not more than 32 mmHg. The force to be applied by artificial means to the crown of a tooth in order to produce such a pressure on the periodontal ligament vessels has not been accurately assessed It is likely to depend on the size and shape of the tooth, and particularly the size and number of the roots. It will also be influenced by other factors, such as the natural forces acting on the teeth and the exact nature and direction of the force applied.

The forces used in successful orthodontic treatment have usually been determined empirically, and no doubt sometimes cause pressures greater than capillary blood pressure.

In considering these forces it is necessary to review the different types of tooth movement which are commonly required.

Types of tooth movement

Several different types of tooth movement occur during orthodontic treatment. Because of the nature of the attachment of the teeth to the alveolar bone all these movements are likely to be complex, but they can be considered in simplified form as follows.
1 Tipping movements.
2 Rotational movements.
3 Bodily movements.
4 Torque movements.
5 Vertical movements.

TIPPING MOVEMENTS

This is perhaps the simplest movement, and the one most readily carried out. Force applied at one point on the crown of a tooth will cause the tooth to tilt away from the force. The centre of rotation of the tooth will depend on the exact point at which the force is applied, becoming nearer to the apex of the root as the point of application becomes nearer to the incisal or occlusal tip of the crown. Christiansen and Burstone (1969) have shown that the amount of force applied does not affect the position of the centre of rotation. In practice, Stephens (1979) has found

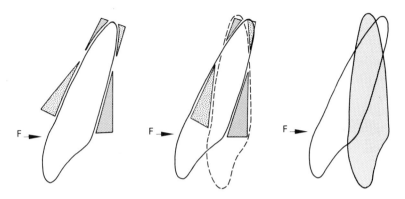

Fig. 9.3. Tipping movement. A force applied to a single point on the crown of the tooth results in bone resorption and deposition to bring about tipping of the tooth. The pressure on the periodontal tissues is greatest near the apex and the cervical margin of the tooth.

that with single rooted teeth the centre of rotation is most frequently located in the middle third of the root (Fig. 9.3).

As tipping movements are readily brought about, the forces required are generally rather less than for some other movements. Crabb and Wilson (1972) found that forces of 0.3 N, 0.4 N and 0.5 N would produce satisfactory distal tipping movement on permanent upper canine teeth, the degree of force not having any material effect on the speed of movement, but the 0.5 N force tended to give rise to more discomfort and difficulty with the appliance. Reitan (1957) found that intermittent forces of 70–100 g (c. 0.7–1.0 N) may produce cell-free areas in the periodontal ligament of an upper canine. Buck and Church (1972) showed that a tipping force of approximately 0.7 N produced undermining resorption on upper premolars.

ROTATIONAL MOVEMENTS

The rotation of a tooth in its socket requires the application of a force couple. This can be produced either by applying a force to one point of the crown and a 'stop' to prevent movement of other parts of the crown, or more efficiently by applying opposite forces to different areas of the tooth (Fig. 9.4). The cross-sectional form of the root will obviously have an important bearing on the ease with which rotational movements are accomplished.

Rotational movements do not normally require any greater force than tipping movements, but there is a much greater tendency for

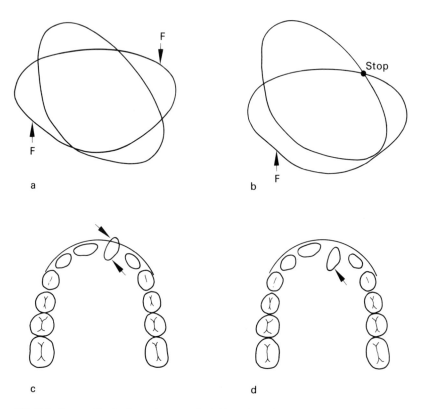

Fig. 9.4. Two methods of rotating a tooth: (a) by using a force couple; (b) by using a single force and a 'stop'. In (a) the centre of rotation is near the centre of the tooth. The situation in (c) would be more appropriate to the use of a force couple, and in (d) to the use of a 'stop'.

rotational movements to relapse. This appears to be due to the fact that although the fibres which attach the tooth to the bone become re-organized fairly quickly during and after tooth movement, the fibres joining the tooth to the gingival tissue remain intact for a long time, simply becoming distorted during tooth movement. In rotational movements most of these gingival fibres are stretched, and this produces the tendency for relapse.

BODILY MOVEMENTS

The term 'bodily movement' is taken to mean the complete translation of a tooth to a new position, all parts of the tooth moving an equal distance. It is difficult to carry out as a single movement, but something

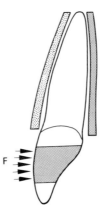

Fig. 9.5. Bodily movement. Force must be applied over a wide area of the crown of the tooth, and there must be provision to prevent tilting. The pressure in the periodontal tissues is evenly distributed.

near to complete bodily movement is possible with appropriate appliances.

As force can only be applied directly to the crown of the tooth, it must be applied over a wide area of the crown, and any tilting movements must be restricted, if bodily movement is to be achieved (Fig. 9.5).

It will be seen from Fig. 9.3 that, in tipping movements, the amount of pressure on the supporting structures is greatest in the areas near the apex and the gingival margins of the root. In bodily movements, however, the pressure is more evenly distributed over the whole length of the supporting structures as shown in Fig. 9.5. Furthermore, for bodily movement to occur, a restraining force must be applied to prevent tilting of the tooth. For these reasons the actual force applied to the crown is usually greater for bodily movements than for tipping movements. Forces of up to approximately 3.0 N have been reported as being successful for bodily movement of upper and lower canines, the actual amount of force depending, of course, on the size of the root. Nikolai (1975) has found that bodily movement of a tooth requires two to three times the force needed for simple tipping of the same tooth, and Quinn and Yoshikawa (1985) have reported that forces of 1.0 N–2.0 N give satisfactory bodily movement of upper canine teeth.

TORQUE MOVEMENTS

The term 'torque' in orthodontic practice is taken to mean the differential movement of one part of a tooth, physically restraining any movement of other parts. It is commonly applied to 'root torque' or

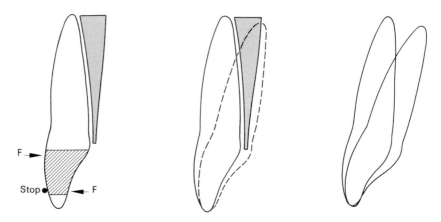

Fig. 9.6. Root torquing movement. A force couple is applied over a wide area of the crown of the tooth, and a stop or opposing force is applied to prevent crown movement. The pressure on the periodontal structures is greatest near the apex of the tooth.

'apical torque', when movement of the root is desired, with little movement of the crown. In this sense it is the opposite of the tipping movement, in which the crown is moved, with little movement of the root. However, as it is not possible to apply direct force to the root of the tooth, root torque is more difficult to achieve than crown movement. At the same time, it is easier to restrain movement of the crown than of the root, and therefore it is theoretically possible to achieve greater differential root movement. The main limitations to root torque lie in the size and form of the bone of the jaw, as the root movement must be confined to the available supporting bone.

Root torque is usually achieved by applying a force couple to the crown of the tooth, at the same time mechanically restricting crown movement in the opposite direction (Fig. 9.6). For practical purposes the forces are generally applied over an area of the crown rather than at single points, this giving greater control over the movements. Fig. 9.6 shows that the pressure on the supporting structures is greatest in the apical area, and the apex of the root moves further than any other part of the tooth. There is a greater risk of apical resorption with this type of movement than with any other type if the forces are not carefully controlled, and the forces required should not be as great as for bodily movement, though they will be greater than for tipping movements because of the necessity of applying an opposing force to restrict movement of the crown. Reitan (1964) reported that a force of approximately 0.5 N is favourable for torquing movement of upper first premolars.

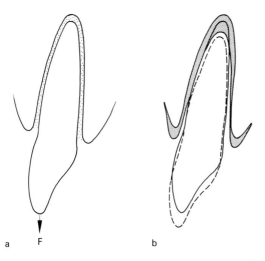

Fig. 9.7. Vertical movement (1). Extrusion. Tension is induced in the supporting structures, and bone deposition is necessary to maintain tooth support.

VERTICAL MOVEMENTS

Vertical movements are essentially bodily movements, but are considered separately because they are easier to produce and involve different types of pressure on the supporting structures.

Extrusion of the tooth from its socket can be achieved without much resorption of bone, bone deposition being required to re-form the supporting mechanism of the tooth (Fig. 9.7) Generally speaking, tension is induced on the whole of the supporting structures, rather than pressure.

Intrusion of the tooth involves resorption of bone, particularly around the apex of the tooth (Fig. 9.8). In this movement the whole of the supporting structures are under pressure, with virtually no areas of tension.

In practice, vertical movements of teeth need the application of force over a wide area of the crown, being difficult to bring about with force applied only to one point. As no counteracting forces are required, forces of the same order as, or less than, those used for tipping movements are sufficient, and, because of the direction of tooth movement, excessive forces are likely to damage the blood vessels entering the dental pulp at the apex, with subsequent death of the tooth. Resorption of the root apices is another potential hazard, particularly with intrusive forces. Dermaut and De Munck (1986) have reported considerable root

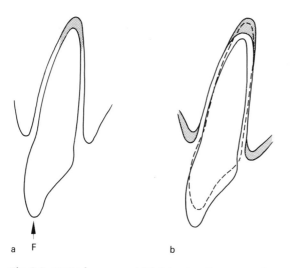

Fig. 9.8. Vertical movement (2). Intrusion. Pressure on the supporting structures is evenly distributed, and bone resorption is necessary, particularly at the apical area and at the alveolar crest.

shortening after intrusion of upper incisors. Reitan (1957) found that a force of approximately 0.25 N was sufficient for the extrusion of an individual tooth, and Burstone (1977) found a similar force suitable for intrusion of an incisor.

MULTIPLE TOOTH MOVEMENT

Orthodontic treatment frequently involves the application of force to move a number of teeth simultaneously. In these circumstances, the total force applied will often exceed the figures previously quoted for individual tooth movement, because the force will be spread over several teeth.

The effects of tooth movement on the dental pulp

Since the main effects of forces applied to the teeth are seen in the periodontal ligament and the surrounding bone, it is generally considered that a healthy periodontal ligament is the only prerequisite for orthodontic tooth movement. Non-vital teeth can be moved, provided there is no periapical infection. However, the dental pulp is not completely unaffected by orthodontic forces. Anstendig and Kronman (1972) have reported consistent disruption of the odontoblast layer in

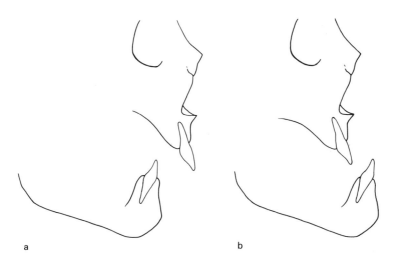

Fig. 9.9. In a very severe skeletal Class 2 (a) or Class 3 (b) relationship it is not possible to overcome the discrepancy of the incisor relationship by tooth movement, because the amount of movement is limited by the size and position of the basal bone of the jaws.

teeth undergoing orthodontic movement and it is possible for teeth to be devitalized by excessive force, though this is uncommon.

Limitations to tooth movement

Teeth under appropriate forces can readily travel through the alveolar bone of the jaws. Limitations to this movement, and therefore limitations to orthodontic treatment, are mainly due to the size and form of the available bone, and to the presence of adverse forces. As the alveolar bone can, to some extent, be reformed to conform to new tooth positions, the bony limitation to tooth movement is the size and form of the basal bone of the jaw. The apex of the tooth must remain on the basal bone, and therefore severe discrepancies in skeletal form, size or relationship cannot be completely overcome by tooth movement. The difficulty of overcoming severe Class 2 and Class 3 skeletal relationships is illustrated in Fig. 9.9. In rather less severe discrepancies, the use of bodily movements or apical torquing movements may overcome the skeletal discrepancy when tipping movements would be insufficient (Fig. 9.10). Fortunately, the very severe skeletal discrepancies are relatively uncommon.

Adverse forces on the teeth, limiting tooth movement, are usually brought about by the oral musculature. It is often possible to overcome

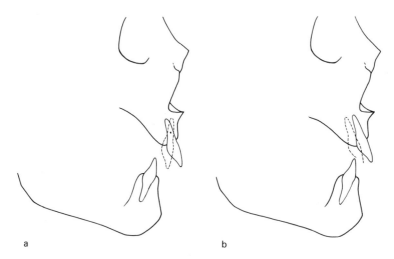

Fig. 9.10. With moderate skeletal discrepancies tipping of the teeth (a) may be insufficient to correct the occlusal relationship, but bodily movement or root torque (b) may bring about a satisfactory improvement.

the forces of the oral muscles during treatment, but if the final position of the teeth at the end of treatment is such that muscular forces are tending to move them towards a different position, then the teeth will move. Therefore, if the tooth position at the end of treatment is to be stable, the muscular forces acting on the teeth must be such as to hold the teeth in their new position. This is usually called a position of 'muscle balance'. Occasionally, the desired tooth position cannot be achieved because it would not be one of 'muscle balance'. This is usually due either to the presence of endogenous tongue thrust, or to adverse lip pressures brought about by skeletal discrepancy.

Retention of tooth position after active treatment

At the end of successful active treatment the teeth should be in a position of 'muscle balance', with all the natural forces acting on them tending to hold them in their new position. It is usually necessary to apply passive mechanical retention at this stage for a period of time. The reason for this is that, at this stage, the supporting structures of the teeth are still undergoing active modification. Bone is being resorbed and deposited in the socket, and in particular the supporting structures of the teeth are under stress. If the teeth are released at this stage the 'recoil' of the supporting structures may be sufficient to overcome any muscular forces acting on the teeth, and partial or complete relapse may occur. In some circumstances, the forces holding the teeth in their new position are sufficient to prevent any relapse, as when an upper incisor has been moved across the lower arch and is held in its new position by the forces of occlusion, but usually a period of retention is necessary. This period of retention varies according to the amount of tooth movement which has been achieved and the type and degree of forces acting on the teeth in their new position. Rotation of teeth needs the longest retention, because in this type of movement all the free gingival fibres are stretched. Perston (1973) has found that the degree of relapse following rotation of teeth is related to the degree of rotation effected, and to the length of passive retention after treatment. Some relapse occurred even after 14 months retention. For most other tooth movements a period of 6 months passive retention is usually sufficient. Pinson and Strahan (1974) have shown that retention time and relapse following rotation can be reduced if pericision—the cutting of the gingival fibres round the tooth—is carried out. Edwards (1988) found significant reduction of relapse using this method, and no detrimental effect on the periodontal condition.

Summary

Tooth movement is the basis of orthodontic treatment.

Experimental work since the early 20th century has led to the 'classical' concept that force on the tooth produces reactions within the periodontal ligament, which lead directly to bone resorption and deposition in the wall of the tooth socket, and consequent tooth movement.

The observed reactions in the ligaments are as follows.

1   Under gentle forces

Hyperaemia; increase in osteoclasts and osteoblasts; direct frontal resorption of bone on the 'pressure' side and deposition of osteoid tissue on the 'tension' side of the socket.

2   Under stronger forces

Ischaemia; reduction of cellular element on the 'pressure' side; endosteal undermining resorption of the socket wall.

3   Under severe forces

Necrosis of periodontal ligament tissue; massive undermining resorption; possibly root resorption and healing by ankylosis.

More recent research has suggested that these reactions may be mediated by factors outside the periodontal ligament, particularly the piezoelectric or mechanochemical effects of stress-deformation of the alveolar bone.

The force necessary for successful tooth movement depends on the type of movement desired, and on the size and shape of the roots.

Types of tooth movement

1 *Tipping movement:* single point application; light force needed.

2 *Rotational movement:* force couple; light force needed.

3 *Bodily movement:* area application with restraint to prevent tipping; greatest force needed.

4 *Torque movement:* area application with restraint of crown movement; intermediate force needed; risk of apical resorption.

5 *Vertical movement:* area application; light force needed; risk of pulpal death.

Limitations to tooth movement are imposed by the size of the dental base and the forces of the oral musculature.

Retention of tooth position is usually needed after tooth movement, particularly after rotations.

References

Anstendig, H. S. & Kronman, J. H. (1972) A histologic study of pulpal reaction to orthodontic tooth movement in dogs. *Angle Orthod*, **42**, 50–55.

Baumrind, S. (1969) A reconsideration of the propriety of the 'pressure-tension' hypothesis. *Am J Orthod*, **55**, 12–22.

Buck, D. L. & Church, D. H. (1972) A histologic study of tooth movement. *Am J Orthod*, **62**, 507–516.

Burstone, C. R. (1977) Deep overbite correction by intrusion. *Am J Orthod*, **72**, 1–22.

Christiansen, R. L. & Burstone, C. J. (1969) Centers of rotation within the periodontal space. *Am J Orthod*, **55**, 353–369.

Cockran, G. V., Pawluk, R. J. & Bassett, C. A. L. (1967) Stress generated electric potentials in the mandible and teeth. *Arch Oral Biol*, **12**, 917–920.

Crabb, J. J. & Wilson, H. J. (1972) The relation between orthodontic spring force and space closure. *Dent Practit*, **22**, 233–240.

Davidovitch, Z., Shanfield, J. L. & Batastini, P. J. (1972) Increased production of cyclic AMP in mechanically stressed alveolar bone in cats. *Eur Orthod Soc Trans*, pp. 477–485.

Dermaut, L. R. & De Munck, A. (1986) Apical root resorption of upper incisors caused by intrusive tooth movement. A radiographic study. *Am J Orthod*, **90**, 321–326.

Edwards, J. G. (1988) A long-term prospective evaluation of the circumferential supracrestal fiberotomy in alleviating orthodontic relapse. *Am J Orthod*, **93**, 380–387.

Epker, B. N. & Frost, H. M. (1965) Correlation of bone resorption and formation with the physical behaviour of loaded bone. *J Dent Res*, **44**, 33–41.

Gianelly, A. A. (1969) Force-induced changes in the vascularity of the periodontal ligament. *Am J Orthod*, **55**, 5–11.

Grimm, F. M. (1972) Bone bending, a feature of orthodontic tooth movement. *Am J Orthod*, **62**, 384–394.

Justus, R. & Luft, J. H. (1970) A mechanochemical hypothesis for bone remodelling induced by mechanical stress. *Calc Tiss Res*, **5**, 222–235.

Khouw, F. E. & Goldberger, P. (1970) Changes in vasculature of the periodontium associated with tooth movement in the rhesus monkey and dog. *Arch Oral Biol*, **15**, 1125–1132.

Mostafa, Y. A., Weakes-Dybuig, M. & Osdoby, P. (1983) Orchestration of tooth movement. *Am J Orthod*, **83**, 245–250.

Nikolai, R. J. (1975) An optimum orthodontic force theory as applied to canine retraction *Am J Orthod*, **68**, 290–302.

Oppenheim, A. (1911) Tissue changes, particularly of the bone, incident to tooth movement. In *Eur Orthod Soc Trans*, pp. 303–359.

Perston, C. M. (1973) Periodic observation of the relapse of upper incisors which had been rotated by an appliance. *J Dent*, **1**, 125–133.

Picton, D. C. A. (1965) On the part played by the socket in tooth support. *Arch Oral Biol*, **10**, 945–955.

Pinson, R. R. and Strahan, J. D. (1974) The effect on the relapse of orthodontically rotated teeth of surgical division of the gingival fibres—pericision. *Br J Orthod*, **1**, 87–91.

Quinn, R. S. & Yoshikawa, D. K. (1985) A reassessment of force magnitude in orthodontics. *Am J Orthod*, **88**, 252–260.

Reitan, K. (1951) The initial tissue reaction incident to orthodontic tooth movement. *Acta Odont Scand*, **9**, Suppl. 6.

Reitan, K. (1957) Some factors determining the evaluation of forces in orthodontics. *Am J Orthod*, **43**, 32–45.

Reitan, K. (1964) Effects of force magnitude and direction of tooth movement on different alveolar types. *Angle Orthod*, **34**, 244–255.

Rygh, P., Bowling, K., Hovlandsdal, L. & Williams, S. (1986) Activation of the vascular system: a main mediator of periodontal fiber remodelling in orthodontic tooth movement. *Am J Orthod*, **89**, 453–468.

Sandstedt, C. (1904) Einige Beiträge zur Theorie der Zahnregulierung. *Nord Tand Tidskr*, **5**, 236.

Sandstedt, C. (1905) Einige Beiträge zur Theorie der Zahnregulierung. *Nord Tand Tidskr*, **6**, 1.

Sandy, J. R. & Harris, M. (1984) Prostaglandins and tooth movement. *Eur J Orthod*, **6**, 175–182.

Schwarz, A. M. (1932) Tissue changes incidental to orthodontic tooth movement. *Int J Orthod*, **18**, 331–352.

Stephens, C. D. (1979) The orthodontic centre of rotation of the maxillary central incisor. *Am·J Orthod*, **76**, 209–217.

Storey, E. (1973) The nature of tooth movement. *Am J Orthod*, **63**, 292–314.

Tanne, K., Saduka, M. & Burstone, C. J. (1987) Three dimensional finite element analysis for stress in the periodontal tissue by orthodontic forces. *Am J Orthod*, **92**, 499–505.

Yamasuki, K., Shibata, Y., Imai, S., Tani, Y., Shibasaki, Y. & Fukuhara, T. (1984) Clinical application of prostaglandin E_1 upon orthodontic tooth movement. *Am J Orthod*, **85**, 508–518.

Zengo, A. N., Pawluk, R. J. & Bassett, C. A. L. (1973) Stress-induced bioelectric potentials in the dento-alveolar complex. *Am J Orthod*, **64**, 17–27.

10

The planning of orthodontic treatment

Orthodontic treatment involves the correction of anomalies of the occlusion and position of the teeth as far as is deemed necessary and possible. To this end, the careful planning of treatment is as important as the actual treatment itself, for unless it is correctly planned the treatment is unlikely to be successful.

Before treatment is planned, there must be adequate assessment of the situation, and the stages of assessment and planning may be considered as follows:

1 Background information.
2 Assessment of occlusal variations.
3 Assessment of aetiological factors and limitations to corrective treatment.
4 Outline of treatment objectives.
5 Detailed treatment plan.

Background information

As with all dental treatment, it is necessary to have a certain amount of information about the patient. Orthodontic treatment cannot be considered in isolation, but must be part of the overall dental care programme. It is necessary to have information on the patient's age and awareness of the problem, any previous dental treatment and attitudes to treatment, and the medical history and state of health. Details of the oral health condition, dietary and oral hygiene habits are also important. If the patient is a child, it is also necessary to ascertain the parents' awareness and attitude to treatment.

All this information has its value. The age of the patient is important in relating general and dental development to chronological age, and in determining growth rate and stage of maturity. It may be important in choosing the best time for treatment. Previous treatment, oral health, attitudes and awareness are all important, though adverse findings in these respects need not contra-indicate orthodontic treatment. Oral health can be improved and attitudes changed, if it is felt necessary. The practicability of doing so must be considered when deciding on orthodontic treatment.

The patient's general health state will occasionally affect decisions on orthodontic treatment. In uncontrolled epilepsy it is undesirable to fit removable appliances. The extraction of teeth or the use of certain appliances may not be advisable in some haemorrhogic diseases. A severely subnormal patient may not be able to manage any appliance. In these and certain other conditions any orthodontic treatment plan may need to be modified or abandoned in the light of the information gained on the general health of the patient.

Assessment of occlusal variations

The nature of all variation from the ideal position and occlusion of the teeth must be assessed. The main sources of variation will be found in the antero-posterior and lateral dental arch relationships, in the vertical incisor relationships, in the crowding or spacing condition of the teeth and in the detail of individual tooth position. Apart from positional variation, these features may bring about variation in occlusal function, which must also be assessed.

The degree of deviation from the ideal is important. Very few individuals show completely ideal occlusal characteristics, but orthodontic treatment may only be needed when the degree of deviation is beyond a certain limit.

Assessment of aetiological factors, and factors limiting treatment

The factors which have brought about the occlusion and position of the teeth must be known in order to have a full understanding of the problem and of the possibilities for treatment. The main aetiological factors, which play a part to some extent in most malocclusions, are the skeletal relationship, the function of the oral musculature and the size of the dentition in relation to the size of the bone of the jaws. Less frequently, local factors such as those discussed in Chapter 7 play a part, either in conjunction with or independent of other aetiological factors.

The importance of assessing the aetiology of the condition lies particularly in deciding the possibilities for treatment. Some factors, if present to a major degree, constitute severe limitations to corrective treatment. Of these, the skeletal relationship and some aspects of oral muscle function are the most important. It may not be possible to overcome the effects of a severe skeletal discrepancy in antero-posterior relationship by orthodontic tooth movement. Similarly, it may not be possible to overcome permanently the effects of endogenous tongue thrust. Therefore the degree of discrepancy in the various aetiological factors must be assessed for successful treatment planning.

It is in this respect that a knowledge of growth changes can be of interest. The degree of discrepancy in aetiological factors may not be constant, and it would be of value in planning treatment to know whether changes are occurring, and whether the changes are favourable or unfavourable. To do this accurately it would be necessary to have records over a period of time, for example, radiographic records which may show that a Class 3 skeletal discrepancy is becoming more severe with growth, or study models which may show the changing effect of tongue or lip activity. It would also be desirable to be able to predict future changes occurring through growth, though individual variation makes this a relatively inaccurate procedure. (see also Chapter 19).

Outline of treatment objectives

Having decided what is wrong, and why it is wrong, it is necessary to outline in broad terms the objectives of orthodontic treatment. In doing this, two considerations must be borne in mind, the *need* for treatment and the *possibilities* for treatment. As has been said previously, few conform to all the ideals with respect to occlusion, but it is not always either necessary or possible to correct every deviation.

The need for treatment must be assessed as discussed in Chapter 8. There will be a good deal of individual variation, and treatment need cannot be assessed entirely on occlusal features. The patient's attitude must be taken into account, particularly in matters associated with personal appearance. In matters of oral health and function the need will be less dependent on the patient's attitude, except at the borderlines of normality.

The possibilities for treatment are limited by the degree of discrepancy of certain aetiological features and by the patient's capacity for cooperation. It is possible with appropriate treatment to correct malocclusion within fairly wide limits, but beyond those limits the skeletal relationship, certain muscular anomalies and some localized tooth malpositions may form barriers to full corrective treatment. It may therefore be necessary to outline treatment objectives which do not aim at correcting every occlusal anomaly which is present. For example, in a very severe Class 2 occlusal relationship with dental arch crowding, it may only be possible to correct the crowding and irregularity of the teeth by orthodontic treatment. The Class 2 relationship may have been brought about by a skeletal discrepancy, the effects of which cannot be overcome by moving the teeth through the bone. The objective of orthodontic treatment in such a situation may be to relieve the crowding and align the teeth within the dental arches, without correcting the antero-posterior relationship. If it is thought necessary to change the skeletal relationship, the possibility of surgical treatment may be explored.

The full co-operation of the patient is essential for successful orthodontic treatment, and the degree of co-operation likely to be achieved must be taken into account in deciding on treatment objectives. Some patients may not be prepared to undergo lengthy and complex treatment, and in such cases it may be reasonable to modify the objectives to fit in with the patient's ability for co-operation.

The importance of setting out the objectives of treatment in broad terms cannot be over-emphasized. A failure to set realistic objectives is one of the main sources of failure of orthodontic treatment. To set realistic objectives means to be aware of all the faults in the occlusion and of the aetiological factors, as well as of the personal factors which affect treatment. It also means being aware of the limits of competence of the operator, because what is a realistic objective for one operator may not be so for another.

Detailed treatment plan

Having decided the objectives of treatment, two basic considerations are required in formulating the detailed treatment plan. These are:
1 The type of tooth movement needed.
2 The space needed for this movement.
The type of tooth movement, as discussed in Chapter 9, will govern the amount of force required for movement and the type of appliance necessary. Tipping movements can usually be carried out by removable appliances, but other types of movement usually need fixed appliances which can apply forces over a wider area of the tooth. In most cases multiple tooth movement is needed, possibly of different types, and all movements necessary must be considered in making the treatment plan.

The space needed for the tooth movement is usually an important consideration. Space is necessary both for the correction of crowding, which is common in many populations, and frequently for the correction of antero-posterior dental arch relationships. Space may also be needed for anchorage purposes for the more difficult tooth movements (see Chapter 12). In some cases, where crowding is the only problem, it is only necessary to make space, and no active tooth movement is needed. More often, irregularities of the teeth need to be corrected by active tooth movement after space has been made.

As the basal bone of the jaw cannot be substantially enlarged by orthodontic treatment, extra space is usually made where necessary by the extraction of teeth. The amount and the position of the space needed must be determined and this will govern the decision on which teeth should be extracted. Other considerations regarding the extraction of teeth in orthodontic treatment will be discussed in Chapter 11.

Following the decision on the type and degree of tooth movement to be carried out, and the space necessary for such movement, it will be necessary to plan the types of appliances, the timing and sequence of the treatment procedures and the type and duration of retention of tooth position. These will all be discussed in later chapters. It is advisable also to make an assessment of the duration of treatment, even though this cannot always be accurate.

A scheme for assessment and treatment planning

With the aforementioned principles in mind, the following outline scheme could be used for the assessment and planning of orthodontic treatment. The various features mentioned will not necessarily be present in every patient, but should be borne in mind as possibilities. In every patient it is necessary to have appropriate radiographs to show the presence and position of unerupted teeth, supernumerary teeth, hypodontia and other dental anomalies. Radiographs to show detail of skeletal form and relationship and incisor inclinations will be valuable in some patients. Dental study models to show tooth position, crowding or spacing condition and occlusal relationships are also essential aids to assessment.

Background information

1   Personal history.
    - Age, sex, residence;
    - reason for attendance;
    - previous dental treatment;
    - attitude to treatment;
    - oral hygiene and dietary habits;
    - thumb or finger sucking habits.

2 General health.
  - Relevant health history;
  - present health state;

Examination of the patient

1 General development—related to age.
2 Speech defects.
3 Oral condition.
  - Oral cleanliness;
  - gingival condition;
  - oral mucous membrane;
  - condition of teeth.
4 Oral muscle form and function.
  - Lips:
    vertical relationship;
    horizontal relationship;
    position at rest—related to teeth;
    function during swallowing and speech.
  - Tongue:
    size;
    position at rest;
    function during swallowing and speech.
  - Summary of the effects of the oral musculature on the occlusion and on treatment.
5 Skeletal relationship—cranio-facial form.
  - Clinical assessment;
  - radiological assessment (where indicated);
  - summary of the effects of the skeletal relationship on the occlusion and on treatment.
6 Position and occlusion of the teeth.
  - teeth present, erupted and unerupted;
  - teeth missing; supernumerary teeth;
  - anterio-posterior dental arch relationship, buccal teeth and incisor teeth (quantity in units or by measurement);
  - incisor inclinations, overjet and overbite;
  - lateral relationships and crossbites;
  - localized tooth malpositions;
  - initial contacts and displacements.
7 Dentition size related to jaw size.

●   Assessment of actual or potential crowding and spacing (quantity in units per quadrant).

Aetiology of the occlusal condition

A summary of the aetiological factors and their possible effects on corrective treatment.
● Muscular factors;
● Skeletal factors;
● Size of the dentition;
● Local factors.

Objectives of orthodontic treatment

A broad outline of objectives.

Treatment plan

● Type and amount of tooth movement.
● Space necessary.
● Extractions: teeth of choice, timing.
● Appliances: stages of treatment.
● Retention.

11

The extraction of teeth in orthodontic treatment

If one subject has caused more controversy than any other in orthodontics, that subject must be the role of extractions in orthodontic treatment. In the past, extraction of teeth has tended to be condemned or acclaimed, according to the fashion of the time or the philosophy of the operator. It has been said that extraction plays no part in orthodontic treatment, on the basis that if crowded teeth are aligned in correct relation to each other, the improved function of the masticatory system will result in growth of the jaws, which in turn will create adequate space for the dentition. Alternatively, it has been said that jaw growth is not dependent on function, and if the jaws are too small to accommodate the teeth, then extraction of teeth will be necessary to relieve crowding and irregularity. There is still difference of opinion regarding the need for extractions, and the difference still centres essentially round the question of function. Functional appliances (see Chapter 15), which work on the principle of utilizing the functional forces of the oral and masticatory musculature, are frequently used successfully, though whether they stimulate jaw growth remains in some doubt. The fact that they are often used without extraction of teeth does not necessarily mean that they provide an alternative to extraction therapy, but more probably that they work best in the patient who does not need extractions.

It is fairly generally accepted in current orthodontic practice that if the jaws are not large enough to accommodate the dentition, there is no satisfactory alternative to extraction. Populations differ in their jaw and dentition sizes, and the prevalence of dental crowding varies in different parts of the world, perhaps in different parts of a country. Therefore, the need for extractions in orthodontic treatment will also vary and this may explain much of the difference of opinion on extraction therapy which has been, and still is prevalent to some extent.

If we accept the premise that the jaws cannot be made larger by functional means, then extraction of teeth in orthodontic treatment will be necessary in two main circumstances.

1 For the relief of crowding.

2 For the correction of antero-posterior dental arch relationship.

Extraction for the relief of crowding

We have already seen (Chapter 6) that the size of the dentition and the size of the basal part of the jaws are to a large extent determined genetically. The size of the dental arch is governed mainly by the basal bone size and the function of the oral musculature. If the dentition is too large to fit in the dental arch without irregularity, it is necessary to reduce the dentition size by extraction of teeth. It is not normally acceptable to increase the size of the dental arch, except in rare circumstances, because the increased dental arch dimensions would not be tolerated by the oral musculature. In those populations therefore, where there is a high prevalence of actual or potential crowding of the teeth, it is frequently necessary to make a decision regarding removal of teeth. Such a decision will be governed by the following considerations:

1   The condition of the teeth.
2   The position of the crowding.
3   The position of the teeth.

The condition of the teeth

The condition of the teeth must be taken into account in planning extractions. Fractured teeth, hypoplastic teeth, grossly carious teeth and teeth with large restorations will all be more favourable for extraction than sound healthy teeth. In assessing condition, the main consideration is the long-term prognosis for the tooth, with the appearance of the tooth being an important secondary consideration. Usually, tooth condition will need to be balanced with other considerations of tooth position in deciding on extractions, and frequently tooth condition is the overriding factor, even when treatment is made more difficult or prolonged by such factors.

The position of the crowding

It is obvious that if crowding is located in one part of the dental arch, it will be more readily corrected if extractions are carried out in that part of the arch, rather than in some more remote uncrowded part. However, this principle is not adhered to absolutely. Crowding of incisors is usually relieved by extraction of premolars, this giving more pleasing final appearance and occlusal balance than removal of incisors. Furthermore, the final tooth position, and particularly the detail of interdental

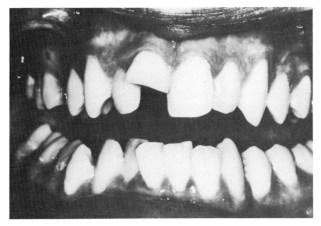

a

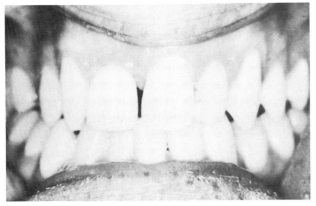

b

Fig. 11.1. (a) Fractured upper central incisor which has moved out of the arch due to lack of lip control. (b) The central incisor has been removed and the lateral incisor moved mesially and crowned.

contacts, must be considered. The first premolar is, in fact, the tooth most commonly removed for the relief of crowding. Being positioned in the centre of each quadrant of the arch, the first premolar is usually near the crowding, whether in the anterior or the buccal segments.

The position of the teeth

The third main consideration is the position of the teeth themselves. Teeth which are grossly malpositioned, and which would be difficult to align, are often the teeth of choice for extraction. In particular, the position of the apex of the tooth must be considered, as it is usually more difficult to move the apex than to move the crown.

Any tooth can be removed to relieve crowding, but some are usually more favourable than others. The following are considerations to be made in extraction of the various individual components of the dentition.

UPPER INCISORS

Upper central incisors are rarely extracted for the relief of crowding, unless their condition is the overriding factor, as when they are severely fractured. In such cases the lateral incisor may be aligned and crowned to simulate the missing central incisor in favourable circumstances (Fig. 11.1).

The usual reasons for removing upper lateral incisors are:

1 Severe malposition of the tooth, particularly when its apex is positioned palatally.

2 Malformation of the tooth, the most common being the coniform crown.

It is also sometimes removed in order to accommodate the canine, when the latter is crowded buccally out of the arch (Fig. 11.2).

LOWER INCISORS

It is often very tempting to extract a lower incisor to relieve crowding, particularly when crowding is confined to the anterior segment of the dental arch. However, generally speaking the results of lower incisor extraction are disappointing, except in certain special circumstances. There is a tendency, after lower incisor extraction, for the remaining anterior teeth to imbricate, and although crowding may be relieved in the short term, forward movement of the buccal teeth leaves the incisor contacts and positions less than ideal (Fig. 11.3).

The two circumstances when extraction of a lower incisor may be indicated, apart from considerations regarding the condition of the teeth, are:

1 When an incisor is completely excluded from the arch (Fig. 11.4).

2 When the lower canines have a marked distal inclination (Fig. 11.5).

In the latter case, removal of a tooth mesial to the canine facilitates its alignment, because crown movement is more readily brought about than apical movement. Even in these circumstances the removal of

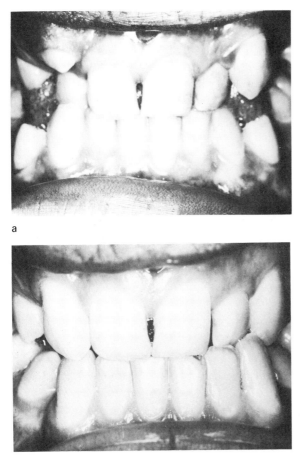

a

b

Fig. 11.2. (a) The right upper lateral incisor is malpositioned and there is insufficient space for the canine to erupt in the arch. (b) The lateral incisor has been removed and has been replaced by the erupting canine tooth.

premolars and alignment of the anterior teeth with appliance therapy is often more suitable.

CANINES

The upper canine is normally removed only when it is severely malpositioned. This may be a developmental malposition, as discussed in Chapter 7, or a malposition due to crowding. The position of the apex is the prime consideration. The canine is a large tooth, and its removal creates more space than the removal of either a lateral incisor or a

a   b

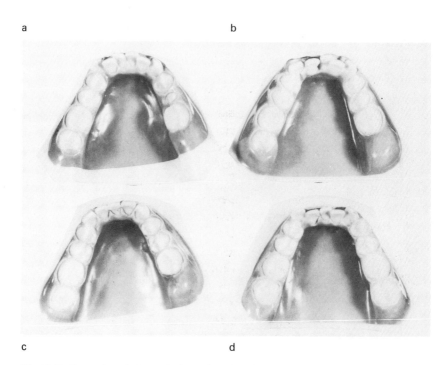

c   d

Fig. 11.3. Extraction of a lower incisor. The original crowding at (a) was relieved by the extraction of an incisor, and the arch was well aligned at (c). Later, however, further overlapping of the remaining teeth developed (d).

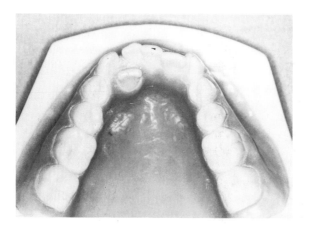

Fig. 11.4. Lower incisor completely excluded from the arch. Removal of this tooth is unlikely to have an adverse effect on the position of the remaining teeth.

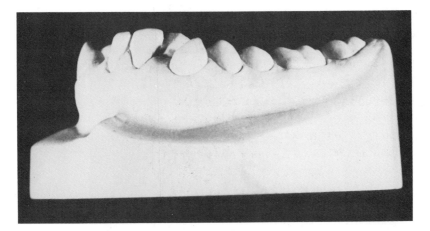

Fig. 11.5. Distal inclination of a lower canine tooth. The removal of an incisor in this circumstance may facilitate alignment of the canine.

premolar. From the point of view of appearance, the canine can be adequately replaced by the first premolar, provided the latter tooth is in good position and not rotated (Fig. 11.6).

Removal of a lower canine should only be considered if the tooth is likely to be very difficult to align. This is usually when it is excluded from the dental arch and the apex is severely malpositioned. The lower lateral incisor—first premolar contact is often poor, and a source of gingival inflammation, and periodontal disease.

FIRST PREMOLAR

As has been mentioned, the first premolar is the tooth most commonly removed for the relief of crowding. It is positioned near the centre of each quadrant of the dental arch, and is therefore normally near the site of crowding. Another important factor is that it can be replaced by the second premolar, which is much the same shape, and which makes a similar contact with the canine. Thus, the loss of the first premolar need not affect the quality of the contacts between the teeth.

SECOND PREMOLAR

Removal of the second premolar for the relief of crowding is usually undertaken when the tooth is itself malpositioned through crowding. As it erupts after the first premolar and first permanent molar, it may be

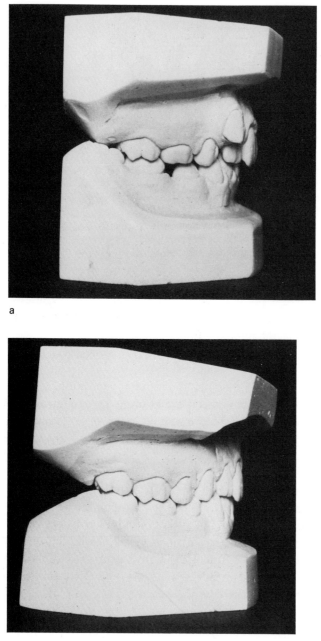

Fig. 11.6. A malpositioned upper canine (a) has been removed and is replaced by the first premolar (b). The lower first premolar has also been removed.

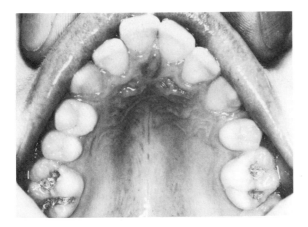

Fig. 11.7. Poor contact between first permanent molar and first premolar following loss of the second premolar.

completely excluded from the dental arch. If removed, it can be satis-factorily replaced by the first premolar unless the first permanent molar has tilted or rotated forward, in which case the contact between the two teeth will not be correct (Fig. 11.7).

FIRST PERMANENT MOLARS

The first permanent molar has been the subject of considerable debate and difference of opinion as to its value in the dental arch, particularly as in the past it has been the most caries-susceptible permanent tooth in childhood. It has been said that it is the keystone of the arch, and should never be removed; alternatively, it has been advocated that the first permanent molars can be removed as a routine measure, with benefit to the dental arches in many cases. These two opposing views cannot both be correct, and it is likely that, with the wide range of variation of occlusal conditions which exists, no single rule regarding the first molar can be made which fits every individual. As with all other teeth, the situation must be viewed on its merits. A reasonable way of considering it is to examine the likely results of removing the first permanent molar.

Extraction before the eruption of the second molar

In this situation, the second molar is likely to move forward as it erupts, particularly in a crowded dentition, tending to take up the position of the extracted first molar.

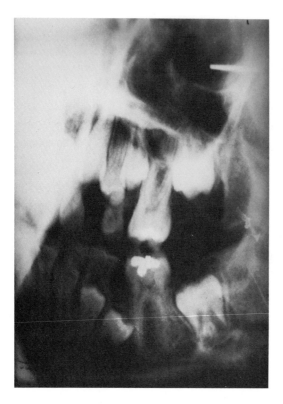

Fig. 11.8. Impaction of lower second premolar against first permanent molar. In such a circumstance it may be desirable to remove the first molar.

Extraction after the eruption of the second molar

In this situation, the second molar will tend to tilt or rotate forward into the first molar space, but can readily be held back if necessary by mechanical means.

With these facts in mind, the removal of the first permanent molars to relieve crowding can be considered as follows:

The first molar is rarely the tooth of choice for extraction to relieve crowding. This is because the contact achieved between the second premolar and second molar is not good, the latter tooth being a different shape from the first molar. The possible exception to this general rule is when the second premolar is unerupted and impacted distally against the first molar, and it is not considered desirable to remove the unerupted premolar (Fig. 11.8).

The first molar, however, is often chosen for extraction if its condition is poor. In this case, there are two general rules for guidance to the best time for extraction.

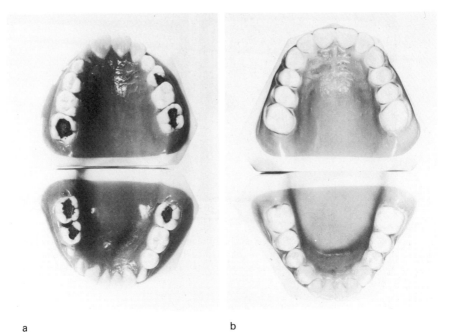

a   b

Fig. 11.9. Removal of first permanent molars before the second molars erupt. (a) The first molars are in poor condition. There is no crowding and no space is needed for reduction of the overjet. The first molars were removed at this stage. (b) The second molars moved forward during eruption to replace the first molars.

1   When crowding is absent, or is confined to the premolar segments, and no space is needed for alignment of anterior teeth.

In this condition, it is usual to remove the first molars before the second molars erupt, so that they will move forward during eruption and take up the first molar positions, the premolar crowding having previously been corrected (Fig. 11.9). In practice, the lower first molars usually need to be removed earlier than the upper first molars, because the second molars travel forward less readily in the lower jaw.

2   When space is required for alignment of anterior teeth. In this condition, the space created by removal of the first molars will usually be needed for alignment of the anterior teeth. Therefore it is necessary to wait for the eruption of the second molars before extracting the first molars, so that space closure by the forward movement of the second molars can be prevented (Fig. 11.10).

In very crowded dentitions, if the first molars are in poor condition, it is sometimes necessary to remove these teeth early, to allow the space to close, and then to remove a premolar from each quadrant for further relief of crowding.

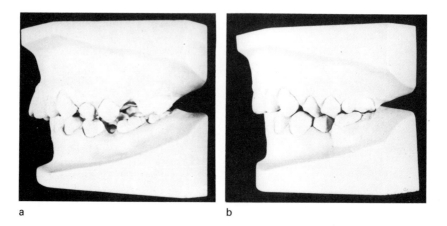

a   b

Fig. 11.10. Removal of first permanent molars after the second molars erupt. (a) The first molars are in poor condition, but there is an excessive overjet. The second molars have erupted. (b) The first molars have been removed, and the space used for reduction of the overjet.

The problems associated with removal of first permanent molars are likely to diminish as more emphasis is placed on the prevention of dental disease, and dental caries less frequently dictates the course of action.

SECOND PERMANENT MOLAR

The second permanent molar is not often removed for the relief of crowding. Its position at the end of the dental arch in childhood means that it is usually remote from the site of crowding, and is not itself actually malpositioned through crowding. However, Richardson (1983) has reported a clinical study in which the extraction of lower second molars resulted in a reduction in lower anterior crowding. The lower second molar is sometimes removed when the first permanent molars have moved forward, leaving insufficient space for eruption of the second premolars. In such cases removal of the second molar will allow distal movement of the first molar to increase the premolar space. It is possible to create space for teeth further forward than premolars in this way, but the amount of tooth movement involved makes this an infrequent choice of treatment.

In removing the second molar, the eventual position of the third molar, if present, must be considered. Removal of the second molar has indeed been advocated for the prevention of lower third molar impaction, but this line of treatment certainly cannot be applied universally. It has been suggested that the only conditions in which lower second molar extraction can result in a reasonable lower third molar position are:

1 When the third molar is upright, or not tilted mesially more than 30°.
2 When the extraction is carried out when only the third molar crown is calcified (Fig. 11.11).

Huggins and McBride (1978) have found a mesial tilt of the third molar of not more than 30° is necessary for a good final position, while Lawlor (1978) maintains that a lack of root formation on the third molar and space between the second and third molar at the time of extraction of the second molar both lead to poor final positioning of the lower third molar. Clinical experience suggests that the latter point is very important, but Dacre (1987) has reported that even in apparently favourable conditions of angulation and crown formation prediction of lower third molar position following the extraction of second molars is uncertain.

In the upper arch, second molar extraction, if carried out before the eruption of the third molar, more often results in satisfactory third molar position, because of the longer eruptive path of the upper third molar.

THIRD PERMANENT MOLARS

Removal of the third molars to prevent or relieve impaction is very frequently carried out. Third molar extraction to prevent crowding of other teeth is also sometimes practised. Progressive crowding of anterior teeth in adolescence and early adult life is not uncommon. It has been suggested that this is due to pressure from erupting teeth at the back of the arches. On the other hand, it may be due to growth changes and changes in muscle activity, causing the dental arches to alter in size or shape but without reduction in size of the dentition. The studies of Richardson (1979) tend to support the forward pressure theory, since there was no evidence of change in incisal angulation in cases of later incisor crowding.

The role of third molar extraction in preventing such crowding is not completely understood. Many clinicians believe that the removal of teeth is likely to have some beneficial effect, but Lindqvist and Thilander (1982) found that it was not possible to predict the effects of third molar extraction on anterior crowding.

Timing of extractions

The correct timing of extractions for the relief of crowding is almost as important as the decision on which teeth should be removed. Generally

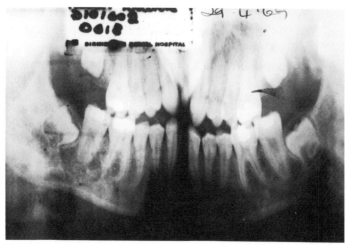

a

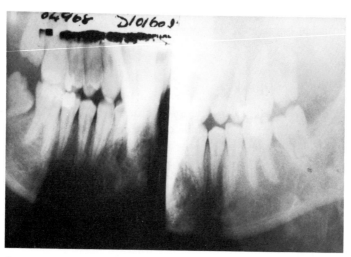

b

Fig. 11.11. Removal of the second molar to prevent third molar impaction. The conditions were more favourable, and the procedure has been more successful, on the right side than on the left.

speaking, it is unwise to remove teeth before they erupt in order to make space for other teeth. The reason for this is that there is a strong tendency in a crowded dentition for teeth to move into any space created by extraction. The removal of unerupted teeth may result in movement of other unerupted teeth, and little space is gained from the extractions. The use of mechanical space maintainers to prevent forward movement is more difficult and needs to be more prolonged in these circumstances than if teeth are allowed to erupt before extractions. The exceptions to this general rule are when the teeth to be removed are the only teeth affected by the crowding or when unerupted teeth are impacted against each other and one must be removed to allow the other to erupt.

A tooth will usually move spontaneously into position more favourably when space is made before it erupts than when it is allowed to erupt before adequate space is made. This principle is commonly employed when providing space for upper canine teeth by removal of first premolars.

Extraction of teeth in the mixed dentition

As has been outlined in Chapter 3, dental arch crowding is a common feature in many populations, and is usually first manifested in the incisor region in the mixed dentition phase. It often seems desirable to begin the correction of crowding during the mixed dentition phase and a system of treatment for such correction, known as *serial extraction*, has been widely practised. The aim of serial extraction is to provide space for the teeth to erupt into good alignment, rather than allow them to erupt into irregular positions in a crowded dentition and subsequently make space and correct the irregularities.

The two basic stages of the procedure are as follows.

1 Removal of the primary canines to make space for the permanent lateral incisors to erupt. The permanent lateral incisors will then take up some of the space which should be available for the permanent canines.
2 Removal of the first premolars to make space for the permanent canines to erupt.

Some operators precede the second stage by removing the first primary molars, on the assumption that this may facilitate the eruption of the first premolars. Kerr (1980) has shown that early loss of primary teeth usually promotes early eruption of permanent successors unless there is space loss.

Thus, if the procedure goes well, the dentition will be reduced by one permanent tooth from each quadrant and the teeth will erupt without irregularity (Fig. 11.12).

While serial extraction can be a useful procedure when conditions are favourable, it is important to appreciate the possible pitfalls in its use and to recognize the conditions in which it will work best.

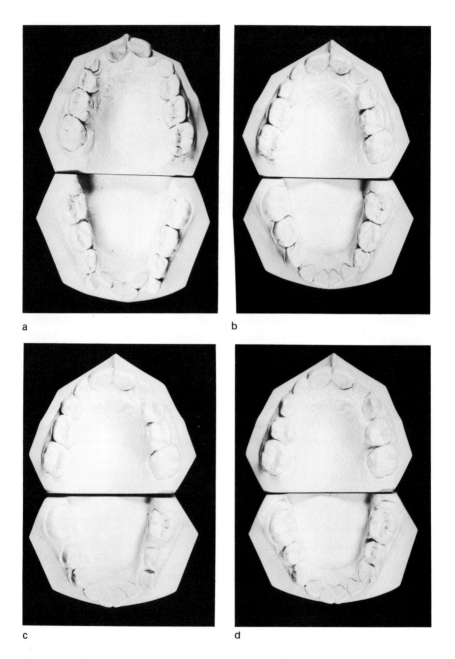

Fig. 11.12. The classical serial extraction procedure. (a) Slight crowding potential in the incisor regions. The primary canines are removed at this stage. (b) Spontaneous alignment of the incisors. (c) Eruption of the first premolars, leaving insufficient space for the upper canines and the lower second premolars. The first premolars are removed at this stage, and space maintainers applied if necessary. (d) Eruption of the canines and second premolars.

Adverse conditions for serial extraction

Too much crowding

Serial extraction works best in conditions of mild to moderate crowding potential. A successful outcome depends on the spontaneous alignment of the permanent incisor teeth before the spaces made by the extraction of the primary canine teeth have closed. Once the permanent incisors have aligned, all residual space can close without detriment, since the ultimate permanent buccal teeth, i.e. the canine and second premolar, will usually occupy slightly less space than the first and second primary molars. In conditions of more severe crowding the first extraction space tends to close before full alignment of the permanent incisors, unless artificial space maintainers are used.

Failure of spontaneous alignment of the permanent incisors

If incisors fail to align spontaneously, then serial extraction in its pure form also fails, although it can be rescued by the use of active appliance treatment. Incisors which are locked by opposing teeth, are severely rotated or whose apices are markedly malpositioned will not align spontaneously, and this should be recognized when planning treatment (Fig. 11.13). Similarly, teeth which are malformed, missing or whose eruption is delayed will jeopardize the success of the procedure.

The indications for serial extraction can be summarized as follows.
1   Mild crowding, manifested by a deficiency of space for the permanent lateral incisors to erupt.
2   No discrepancy in the dental arch relationship. This is not an absolute prerequisite, but the correction of dental arch relationship usually requires the provision of extra space in the arch, and the risk of space loss during serial extraction makes it more suitable for Class 1 occlusions.
3   All teeth present, in good condition and in correct eruptive positions.
4   No occlusal interlocking, severe rotations or apical malpositions of the incisors unless active appliance treatment is available.

The sequence of tooth eruption usually makes serial extraction more successful in the upper arch than in the lower. The upper first premolar erupts, and can be removed, before the upper canine erupts. The lower canine, however, normally erupts before the first premolar, and may be displaced before adequate space can be made. Nevertheless, serial extraction is a useful procedure in a limited number of patients provided careful assessment is made, space loss is prevented, and active appliance treatment is available if necessary.

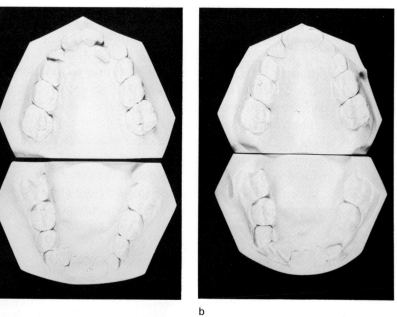

a

b

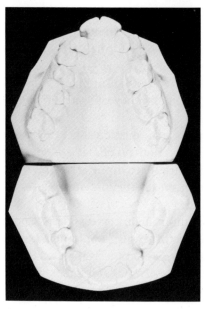

c

Fig. 11.13. Serial extraction complicated by irregularity of the teeth. There is still the need for active appliance treatment.

Extractions for alteration of dental arch relationship

Quite apart from the need for relief of crowding, it is frequently necessary to remove teeth to give space for correction of discrepancies in arch relationship. This applies particularly in the Class 2 relationship, when the upper arch is too far forward in relation to the lower. The upper arch, or more often the anterior segment of the arch, is usually moved back in the course of treatment, and unless the arch is spaced this backward movement can only be made if teeth are removed to provide space.

The factors which govern the decision on which teeth to remove are much the same as for extractions for the relief of crowding, and again the first premolars are the teeth most commonly removed. The detail of how the extraction spaces are used in treatment will be dealt with in a later chapter.

It will be apparent that if there is a discrepancy in the antero-posterior arch relationship which needs correction, and superimposed on this is crowding of the teeth, the need for space is even greater than in either of these conditions separately. Occasionally, more than one tooth needs to be removed from each side of the arch which is to be reduced (Fig. 11.14).

Balancing extractions

If a tooth is removed from one side of a dental arch which is crowded, or which has complete contact of teeth all round, there is a tendency for the remaining teeth to move towards the extraction space. The greatest movement will be forward movement of the teeth behind the space, but there may be some movement of the anterior teeth across the centre of the arch, with subsequent asymmetry, particularly in a crowded arch (Fig. 11.15). It is usual to balance extractions, that is to extract symmetrically on each side of the arch, in order to prevent such lateral asymmetry. It is not necessary to extract the same tooth on each side, merely to provide space on each side.

Balancing extractions are not necessary if the dental arch is spaced, there being no tendency for lateral movement.

Compensating extractions, that is extraction of teeth in opposite jaws, is usually linked to orthodontic appliance treatment. In a Class 1 occlusion with crowding, in some circumstances extraction of teeth is the only treatment needed. In such a case, the arches being equal sizes, it would normally be necessary to extract in both arches, the extractions

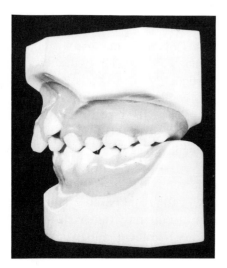

Fig. 11.14. Crowding and Class 2 relationship of the dental arches. It is necessary to make space to relieve the crowding, and more space is required in the upper arch to reduce the overjet.

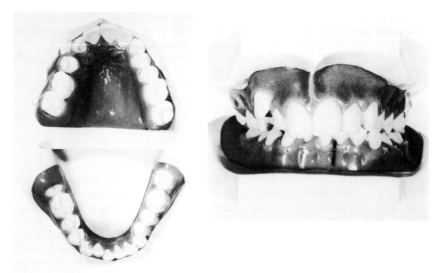

Fig. 11.15. Asymmetry of the dental arches resulting from unbalanced extractions. A tooth has been lost from the upper right quadrant and there is deviation of the upper arch to the right.

being balanced to maintain lateral symmetry, i.e. a tooth (or teeth) would need to be removed from all four quadrants of the jaws. In a Class 2 or Class 3 occlusion extractions would be combined with active appliance treatment if the occlusal discrepancy was to be corrected, and the question of compensating extractions in such situations will be dealt with in later chapters.

Summary

Extraction of teeth is usually carried out for two main reasons.
1 The relief of crowding.
2 To give space for correction of antero-posterior arch discrepancies.

Considerations in the decision on extractions

1 Condition of the teeth.
2 Position of the crowding.
3 Position of the teeth.

Considerations on individual teeth

1 *Upper incisors and canines*—usually removed only if damaged or severely malpositioned.
2 *Lower incisors and canines*—extraction usually best avoided, unless the tooth is excluded from the arch or the canines have a severe distal inclination.
3 *First premolars*—the teeth most commonly extracted. Readily replaced by second premolars, and being in the centre of each quadrant they are usually near the site of crowding.
4 *Second premolars*—usually extracted only if malpositioned. Satisfactorily replaced by first premolars, unless the first molar tilts or rotates.
5 *First molars*—not usually the tooth of choice for extraction. If extraction is necessary due to caries, two general circumstances exist which govern the timing of the extraction.
    ● If no space is needed for alignment of the anterior segment, extract before the second molar erupts.
    ● If space is needed for alignment of the anterior segment, extract after the second molar erupts.
6 *Second molars*—extraction does not allow much spontaneous relief of crowding, but may relieve third molar impaction if:
    ● The third molar is not severely inclined mesially.
    ● The third molar development has not proceeded beyond calcification of the crown at the time of extraction.
7 *Third molars*—sometimes extracted early, though doubt exists as to

whether extraction contributes to relief or prevention of anterior crowding.

Extraction in the mixed dentition: serial extraction

1   Objective. To provide space in a crowded arch as the teeth erupt.
2   Indications
   • Class 1 occlusion.
   • Slight crowding, manifested as a lack of space for the permanent lateral incisor.
   • All teeth present and in correct eruptive positions and good condition.
   • No severe rotations or apical malposition of incisors or interlocking of occlusion.
3   Procedure
   • Extract the primary canines to make space for the permanent lateral incisors.
   • Extract the first premolars, when erupted, to make space for the permanent canines.
4   Potential problems
   • Possible loss of space, making the crowding worse; there may still be irregularity of teeth which needs correction.

Balancing extractions

Lateral symmetry of extraction is necessary in a full or crowded arch to avoid movement of teeth across the centre.

References

Dacre, J. T. (1987) The criteria for lower second molar extraction. *Br J Orthod*, **14**, 1–9.

Huggins, D. G. & McBride, C. J. (1978) The eruption of lower third molars following the loss of lower second molars: a longitudinal cephalometric study. *Br J Orthod*, **5**, 13–20.

Kerr, W. J. S. (1980) The effect of the premature loss of deciduous canines and molars on the eruption of their successors. *Eur J Orthod*, **2**, 123–128.

Lawlor, J. (1978) The effects on the lower third molar of the extraction of the lower second molar. *Br J Orthod*, **5**, 99–103.

Lindqvist, B. & Thilander, B. (1982) Extraction of third molars in cases of anticipated crowding of the lower jaw. *Am J Orthod*, **81**, 130–139.

Richardson, M. E. (1979) Late lower arch crowding: facial growth or forward drift? *Eur J Orthod*, **1**, 219–225.

Richardson, M. E. (1983) The effect of lower second molar extraction on late lower arch crowding. *Angle Orthod*, **53**, 25–28.

12

Principles of orthodontic appliances

Orthodontic appliances fall into two broad categories.

1 Passive appliances which maintain the position of the teeth. These are commonly used for space maintenance after extractions, or for the maintenance of tooth position after active tooth movement.

2 Active appliances which bring about movement of the teeth. These may either incorporate active forces within the appliance, or transmit forces from another source, usually the muscles of mastication or the circumoral musculature.

Appliances may be fixed to the teeth or may be removable by the patient, or may contain a combination of fixed and removable components.

All appliances should be comfortable to wear and readily acceptable by the patient. They should be well tolerated by the oral tissues, and should be sufficiently robust to stand up to the stresses of oral function. They should also be readily cleanable by the patient so that they do not constitute a hazard to oral health. They should be capable of being firmly positioned in the mouth, with no tendency to be inadvertently dislodged, a quality usually known as *retention* or *fixation*.

Active appliances need certain other qualities because of their need to produce tooth movement. These are known as *force* and *anchorage* components.

Force component

The force which brings about tooth movement can be provided in several ways. The following principles are commonly used.

DEFORMATION OF ELASTIC COMPONENTS

Any component of an appliance which can be deliberately deformed and which will tend to return to its original form can be used to apply force to the teeth. In practice, two types of material are used for this purpose, stainless steel wire in the form of springs or arches and natural rubber elastic or similar synthetic compounds.

Stainless steel wire incorporated in removable appliances (Fig. 12.1) or in fixed appliances (see Fig. 14.8) is the most frequently used force

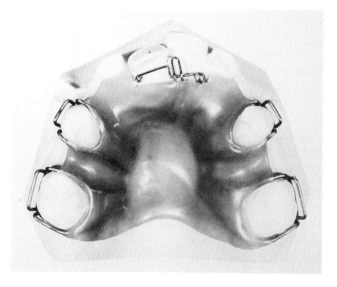

Fig. 12.1. Stainless steel spring in a removable orthodontic appliance to procline an upper central incisor.

component, being readily formed, fairly robust and capable of precise regulation.

Latex rubber elastic or similar compounds can be added to appliances and the elastic force provided will readily bring about tooth movement. Again, such components are used in removable appliances (Fig. 12.2) and in fixed appliances (Fig. 12.3), and also form the basis of extra-oral traction (see Fig. 12.9), which applies force to the teeth from a site outside the mouth.

PROGRESSIVE CHANGE IN THE FORM OF THE APPLIANCE

An appliance which fits closely against the teeth and which can be progressively slightly altered in form can be made to apply a moving force to the teeth. A common example of the use of this principle is the incorporation of a screw between two parts of an appliance (Fig. 12.4). Turning the screw at intervals alters the form of the appliance, and, provided the alteration is not made too quickly, the teeth move in response to the forces applied. The force is intermittent, unlike the more constant force applied by elastic deformation, but with correct use there is no apparent clinical difference in the response.

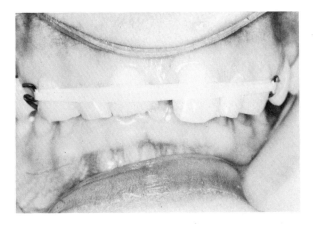

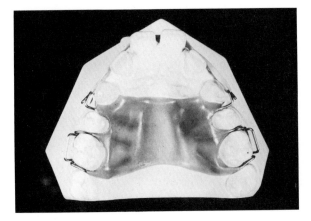

Fig. 12.2. Latex rubber elastic used to retrocline upper incisor teeth in a removable orthodontic appliance.

THE USE OF MUSCULAR FORCES

An orthodontic appliance can be used as a static component in a system which transmits muscular forces to the teeth. In such a system the appliance itself has no built-in force component, but is constructed so that functional muscular behaviour brings about tooth movement. Such appliances are known as *functional appliances,* and will be considered in Chapter 15.

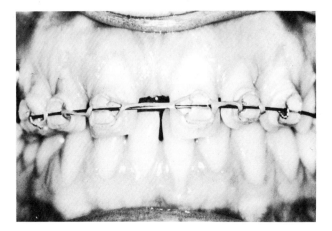

Fig. 12.3. Elastic ligatures used to apply force to the teeth in a fixed appliance.

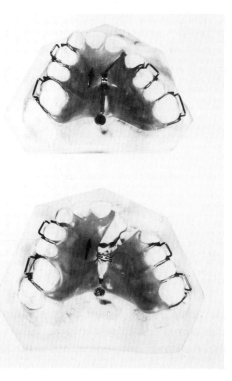

Fig. 12.4. Removable appliance incorporating a screw to widen the dental arch of a patient with cleft palate. The hinge at the back of the appliance allows differential opening.

Anchorage component

The force which moves the teeth must have a basis from which it acts. The base from which the moving force is applied is known as the anchorage, and anchorage is a very important quality of an active appliance. Mechanical principles dictate that the force applied to move the teeth necessitates an equal and opposite force being applied to the anchorage. Frequently, in orthodontic treatment, the anchorage itself consists of teeth, which are, of course, liable to move under the influence of the equal and opposite force. The anchorage of an appliance must therefore be carefully designed so that no undesirable tooth movement occurs.

There are many ways of providing adequate anchorage, and they can be grouped as follows.

SIMPLE ANCHORAGE

This is gained by using teeth, whose movement is not desired, to take the load of the anchorage forces. Since, in this case, the anchor teeth are liable to move, it is necessary to spread the load around as many anchor teeth as possible, so that the force on any one tooth is insufficient to cause movement. In practice, if the anchorage is designed so that less than 0.1 N force is applied to each anchor tooth, little or no movement of the anchor teeth will occur since this appears to be the minimum force for tooth movement (Bass & Stevens 1970). The amount of force on each anchor tooth in simple anchorage is equal to the total moving force component of the appliance divided by the number of anchor teeth (Fig. 12.5).

Simple anchorage is frequently used, and is perfectly satisfactory for many stages of treatment.

RECIPROCAL ANCHORAGE

In some treatment procedures it is desirable to move teeth or groups of teeth in opposite directions. In such cases it is possible to utilize anchorage forces as moving forces, as illustrated in Figs. 12.3 and 13.5.

A frequently used form of reciprocal anchorage is known as *intermaxillary traction,* (Fig. 12.6) in which the forces used to move the whole or part of one dental arch in one direction are anchored by equal forces moving the opposing arch in the opposite direction, thus correcting discrepancies in dental arch relationship.

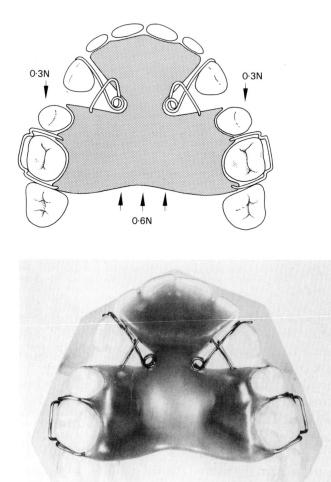

Fig. 12.5. Simple anchorage. A total force of 0.6 N applied to the canine teeth produces an equal and opposite force distributed around the other eight teeth, i.e. a force of less than 0.1 N on each anchor tooth. The anchor teeth are unlikely to move under this force.

REINFORCING ANCHORAGE

It frequently happens that the teeth available for simple anchorage are not sufficient in number or in size to resist the forces necessary for treatment, and that reciprocal anchorage is not appropriate to the type of treatment to be carried out. In such circumstances it is necessary to reinforce the anchorage to avoid unwanted movements of the anchor

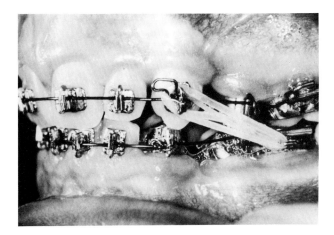

Fig. 12.6. Intermaxillary traction. The elastic force moves the upper anterior teeth back and the lower posterior teeth forward, using reciprocal anchorage.

teeth. Anchorage can be reinforced by making movement of the anchor teeth more difficult or by adding extra anchorage forces from other sites. Bodily movement of the teeth requires greater force than tipping movement. Therefore, if the anchor teeth can be held so that they cannot tilt, but can only move bodily, they are more resistant to the anchorage forces. Banding the anchor teeth prevents tipping, and therefore reinforces anchorage. This is the basis of the labio-lingual appliance system (Chapter 14). Similarly, joining together posterior anchor teeth on opposite sides of the arch helps to prevent their movement, particularly in V-shaped arches. With removable appliances, a closely fitting archwire round some of the anchor teeth helps to prevent tipping, and improves anchorage (Fig. 12.7).

Extra-oral forces

Extra forces for either moving the teeth or for anchoring their movement can be obtained from outside the mouth, usually from the cervical or occipital region. These forces provide either extra-oral traction or extra-oral anchorage. The difference between the two lies in the amount of force used. For extra-oral traction, forces sufficient to move the teeth must be applied, and if blocks of teeth or a whole arch are to be moved then the force applied would need to be considerable. Forces of up to 10 N have been recommended for whole arch movement

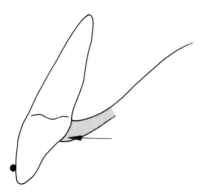

Fig. 12.7. Reinforcing anchorage. The reciprocal force from a removable appliance moving buccal teeth distally tends to tilt incisors forward. A closely fitted archwire helps to prevent tilting and reinforces the anchorage.

(Mills *et al.* 1978). There is some evidence to suggest that such forces act by restraining growth as well as by moving the teeth (Howard 1982). For *extra-oral anchorage*, on the other hand, the active force is incorporated in the intra-oral appliance, and the function of the extra-oral force is to cancel out the reciprocal action of the active force component so that anchor teeth do not move. Since extra-oral appliances are usually worn at least half the time, it is usual to apply a force equal to at least twice the total force incorporated in the intra-oral force component.

There are several systems of application of extra-oral forces. The two which will be described here are the system using a face bow, with the force applied to the posterior teeth, and the system using J hooks, with the force applied to the anterior segment of the arch. Both these systems are used to apply a backward or upward force to the upper dental arch. This is the most common use of extra-oral force. Other systems have been devised to apply a forward force to the upper arch in correction of Class 3 occlusal relationships (Nanda 1980). Extra-oral forces can also be applied to the lower arch (Orton *et al.* 1983).

THE FACE BOW

The face bow for extra-oral force application consists of an intra-oral arch which is attached to the posterior teeth, and an integral extra-oral bow to which the force is applied (Fig. 12.8). In view of their length, these components need to be constructed of fairly thick wire to ensure rigidity. The inner bow is usually made from 1.25 mm, and the outer bow from 1.5 mm stainless steel. The inner bow is attached to the dental arch via a tube on each side, which is either soldered to a molar crib on a removable appliance or to a molar band on a fixed appliance. To prevent

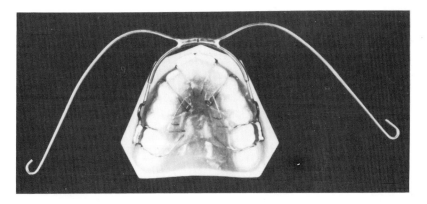

Fig. 12.8. Face bow and intra-oral bow for extra-oral anchorage, attached to a removable appliance via tubes soldered to Adams cribs.

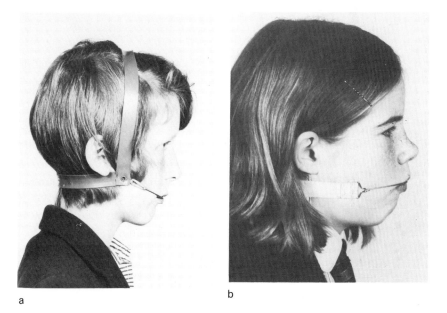

a

b

Fig. 12.9. (a) Headgear with elastics; and (b) elasticated neck band attached to face bow to provide extra-oral force.

the bow sliding too far through the tubes it is usual to incorporate a stop in the form of a loop or bend in the wire, so that the bow remains just clear of the incisor teeth.

The force is applied from a headgear or a neckband, via elastics to the outer bow (Fig. 12.9). A neckband, which is often elasticated tends to

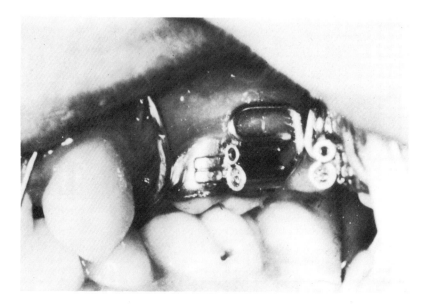

Fig. 12.10. Molar band with tube for extra-oral force via a face bow. Note modified retention loops for the removable appliance.

produce a horizontal or slightly downward pull which may dislodge a removable appliance. This type of cervical traction is therefore better for fixed appliances, which will not be dislodged, and for those movements which require a horizontal backward pull. If removable appliances are to be used cervical traction is better applied via cemented molar bands (Fig. 12.10). With a headgear applying occipital traction the direction of pull can be adjusted to include an upward component (Fig. 12.11).

The amount of force applied can be modified either by adjusting the length of the elasticated neckband or by changing the number or strength of the elastic bands.

J HOOKS

J hooks from an occipital headgear can be used with both removable and fixed appliances. Since the direction of pull always has an upward component this system is particularly useful for reinforcing anchorage in removable appliance treatment (Usiskin & Webb 1972; Quealy & Usiskin 1979).

The J hooks are attached on each side to a headgear, and engage on the anterior segment of the arch (Fig. 12.12). Again, the force comes

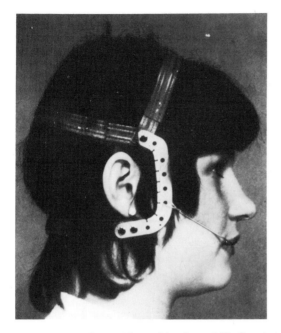

Fig. 12.11. Headgear with provision for variable direction of extra-oral force.

from elastics between the headgear and the hooks, and is readily adjustable. In fixed appliance treatment J hooks can be used directly for the distal movement of individual teeth.

Although they are of great value and are very widely used in orthodontic treatment, it must always be remembered that extra-oral appliances carry some risk of injury to the patient or others unless properly designed and used. In particular, the presence of an extra-oral hook for attaching elastics to the head or cervical gear and the fact that the whole assembly is under elastic tension when in use provides a potential risk of serious injury, even though this risk is very small (Seel 1980; Booth-Mason & Birnie 1988). It is therefore wise to insist on the following precautions when using extra oral forces.

1 Any extra-oral hooks should be as closed as practicable, and aligned vertically. Wire ends should be covered with plastic tubing.

2 The patient should be warned of the risks and instructed to wear the apparatus only during quiet occupation, never during active play. Elastic components should be placed only after the intra-oral part of the apparatus is fitted, and removed before the apparatus is removed from the mouth.

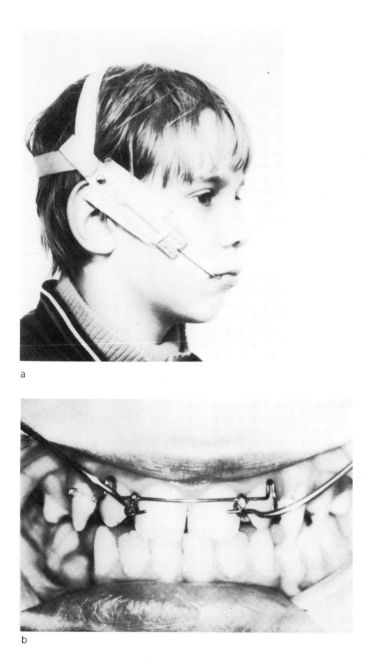

a

b

Fig. 12.12. (a) Occipital headgear for medium — high pull with J hooks. (b) Attachment of J hooks to spurs on labial arch on a removable appliance.

Various 'safety' headgears are now available which reduce, though do not eliminate, the risks.

Apart from the principles mentioned above, most appliances gain some anchorage from other oral soft or hard tissues. Many removable appliances gain anchorage from the hard palate and alveolar structures, and pressures from the lips and tongue can provide some anchorage for certain tooth movements. Generally speaking however, it is best to ignore such additional anchorage in appliance design and to make sure that the anchorage gained from the teeth or from extra-oral structures is sufficient. Many treatments fail through inadequate anchorage. None fail through too much anchorage.

As has been mentioned, all appliances need adequate retention. The provision of firm retention for active appliances is more critical and sometimes more difficult than for passive appliances, since the force component in active appliances not only tends to dislodge the appliance if retention is less than perfect, but also must have a firm base if it is to work to its greatest efficiency.

Summary

Orthodontic appliances may be passive or active, may be fixed to the teeth, removable by the patient, or a combination of fixed and removable components.

All appliances must be comfortable and well tolerated and have adequate retention.

Active appliances must also have a force component and an anchorage component.

Force component

This may be provided by:
1 Deformation of elastic components, usually steel wire or rubber.
2 Progressive change in form of the appliance, usually by means of a screw.
3 The use of muscular forces—functional appliances.
4 The use of extra-oral forces.

Anchorage component

Anchorage is the basis from which the force component is applied.

It can be:

1   Simple anchorage, using teeth to resist the anchor forces.
2   Reciprocal anchorage, where teeth are to be moved in opposite directions, the moving forces providing the anchor forces.

Anchorage can be reinforced by making movement of anchor teeth more difficult, e.g. using bands or close-fitting arches, or by adding extra anchor forces, e.g. extra-oral anchorage.

References

Bass, T. P. & Stevens, C. D. (1970) Some experiments with orthodontic springs. *Dent Practit*, **21**, 21–32.

Booth-Mason, S. & Birnie, D. (1988) Penetrating eye injury from orthodontic headgear—a case report. *Eur J Orthod*, **10**, 111–114.

Howard, R. D. (1982) Skeletal changes with extra-oral traction. *Eur J Orthod*, **4**, 197–202.

Mills, C. M., Holman, R. G. & Graber, T. M. (1978) Heavy intermittent cervical traction in Class II treatment: A longitudinal cephalometric assessment. *Amer J Orthodont*, **74**, 361–379.

Nanda, R. (1980) Biochemical and clinical considerations of a modified protraction headgear. *Am J Orthod*, **78**, 125–129.

Orton, H. S., Sullivan P. G., Battagel, J.M. and Orton, S. (1983) The management of Class III and Class III tendency occlusions using headgear to the mandibular dentition. *Br J Orthodont*, **10**, 2–12.

Quealy, R. & Usiskin, L. (1979) High pull headgear with J hooks to upper removable appliances. *Br J Orthod*, **6**, 41–42.

Usiskin, L. & Webb, W. B. (1972) Extra oral anchorage for upper removable appliances. *Br Dent J*, **133**, 140–145.

Seel, D. (1980) Extra-oral hazards of extra-oral traction. *Br J Orthod*, **7**, 53.

13

Principles of removable appliance treatment

Removable orthodontic appliances are so-called because they are designed to be fitted and removed by the patient. This facility brings with it certain advantages but also some disadvantages, and therefore this type of appliance has limitations in its use, which must be carefully observed in planning treatment.

The main relative advantages of removable appliances can be listed as follows. They may be compared with the other main appliance system, i.e. fixed appliances, which will be considered in the next Chapter.

1 The appliance is removable by the patient and can therefore be readily cleaned. The dentition and oral structures can also be maintained in a clean and healthy state during appliance therapy.

2 It is difficult to apply severely excessive forces to the teeth with removable appliances, such forces being dissipated by dislodgement of the appliance.

3 The construction of removable appliances is mainly carried out in the laboratory, and relatively little surgery time is involved.

The main disadvantages of removable appliances are as follows:

1 They can bring about only a limited type of tooth movement. It will be seen later that on the whole, the removable appliance applies its force to a relatively small area of the crown of the tooth. This brings about a tipping movement, which is the main movement possible with this type of appliance. Rotational movements can also be achieved by using force couples. Bodily movement or apical torquing movement are difficult, if not impossible, and removable appliances are not satisfactory for these types of tooth movement.

2 Anchorage of tooth movement is sometimes difficult, since anchor teeth cannot be prevented from tilting. This is somewhat countered by the fact that only tilting movements are being achieved by the appliance, and these require less force than bodily or torquing movements. Therefore the anchor teeth usually come under less strain than with fixed appliances.

3 Retention of the appliance is more difficult than with fixed appliances.

4 A high degree of co-operation and a certain amount of skill is required from the patient, who has to remove, clean and replace the

appliance at frequent intervals. Co-operation from the patient is necessary for all orthodontic appliance treatment, but skill in removing and replacing the appliance is essential in removable appliance therapy. To fall within the limits of the patient's skill, the appliance must usually be kept relatively simple, and simultaneous multiple tooth movements are therefore more difficult with removable appliances than with fixed appliances.

It will be seen from the above that removable appliances are limited in their scope. They are readily applicable only to patients who can cope with their own role in the treatment, and whose active tooth movement involves only tipping of teeth and limited rotatory movements. Nevertheless, a number of patients fall within this category. Many of the less severe malocclusions can be corrected by utilizing tipping movements and removable appliance therapy plays an important part in orthodontic treatment.

Components of removable appliances

As with all orthodontic appliances, removable appliances must have retention, and if active, must have a force and an anchorage component. There must also be a connecting framework, usually made in acrylic resin.

Retention component

In the past, the difficulty of providing adequate retention has placed severe limitations on the efficiency of active removable appliances. With the development of the modified arrowhead clasp by Adams (1950, 1953, 1984) now usually called the Adams clasp, problems of retention have to a large extent been overcome, provided that appropriate teeth are present for the clasp to be fitted. Originally designed to be made on first permanent molars (Figs. 13.3–13.5), the Adams clasp can be modified for premolars or even incisors, where it gives good retention. It can be used less effectively on second permanent molars, these teeth not being the ideal shape for such purpose.

Other aids to retention of removable appliances are available, various arch wires and clasps being of some help, and muscle pressures, adhesion and tooth undercut areas add a little to retention, but the Adams clasp remains the main retentive device, without which removable appliance therapy would be much less satisfactory.

Force component

The force component in removable appliances is usually provided by means of springs, elastics or screws.

Springs are constructed from stainless steel wire. The most commonly used is the finger spring, which is fixed to the appliance at one end, the free end being used to apply a force to the tooth. The spring is deformed to a passive position some distance from the position of the tooth and, when moved to its active position against the tooth, applies a force. The force is directly proportional to the distance from the passive to the active position of the free end of the spring, and is also proportional to the diameter and inversely proportional to the length of the wire. For a given deflection from passive to active positions, the thicker the wire the greater the force produced, and the longer the wire the less the force produced at the free end. Increasing the length of the wire, however, increases the range of action of the spring, and for this reason it is usual to incorporate a coil in the wire, which effectively increases its length within the limits of the appliance. Bass and Stevens (1970) have investigated certain properties of springs, and have shown:

1 That the direction in which the coil is wound makes little difference to the effectiveness of the spring.

2 That the increase in length of the wire achieved by incorporating a coil increases the flexibility of the spring, though not to the same extent as the same increase in length without incorporating a coil.

3 That a double coil provides further increase in the flexibility of the spring by incorporating more wire in a given length of spring. Similar principles apply to springs of other types.

Some springs commonly used in removable appliances are illustrated in Figs. 12.1, 12.5, 13.3 and 13.5.

Elastics are used less frequently in removable appliances than springs, but can provide the force component in suitable circumstances (see Fig. 12.2). Again, co-operation from the patient is essential, since elastics need to be changed frequently and applied correctly.

Elastics are the usual force component in extra-oral traction (Chapter 12).

Screws of various types are used to provide intermittent forces in removable appliances. They have the advantage that they are easier for the patient to manage than springs, and are therefore useful for the less skilful patient. The screw is adjusted by the patient or parent at intervals, in most cases once or twice a week, but sometimes more frequently. A further advantage of the screw is that it has less tendency

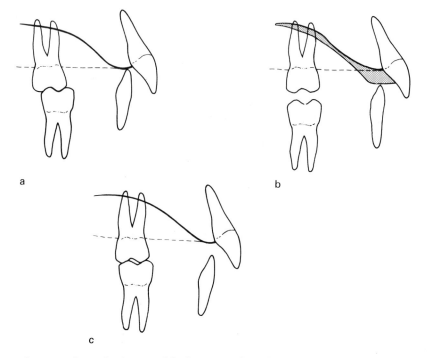

Fig. 13.1. The mode of action of the flat anterior bite plane. (a) The deep incisal overbite with the posterior teeth in occlusion. (b) With the appliance fitted, the lower incisors touch the bite plane and the posterior teeth remain apart. Further vertical development of the lower posterior teeth can take place. (c) When the bite plane is removed, the incisal overbite has been reduced.

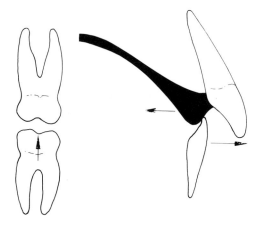

Fig. 13.2. The mode of action of the inclined anterior bite plane. The buccal teeth are kept apart, and further vertical development can occur, thus reducing the incisal overbite. It has also been claimed that the incline of the bite plane induces a forward mandibular posture and reciprocal backward force on the upper appliance from the masticatory forces.

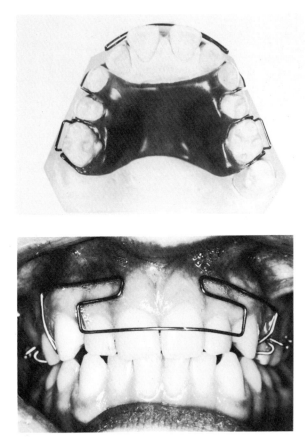

Fig. 13.3. Labial bow to retrocline central incisors. As only two teeth are being moved, anchorage presents little problem.

to dislodge the appliance than springs, and it therefore provides a more stable appliance for moving several adjacent teeth in the same direction. Most screws produce approximately 0.2 mm movement per quarter turn. Experiments have shown that such movement on a rigid appliance can result in grossly excessive forces being applied to the teeth, provided the appliance is not displaced. In practice, it is likely that there is slight displacement of the appliance at every turn of the screw, as well as some deformation of the wire clasps, and thus not all the potential force is applied to the teeth. The amount of force applied to each tooth by a screw appliance will depend on the number of teeth being moved, each tooth receiving its share of the total force.

Anchorage component

The principles of simple and reciprocal anchorage are readily applied to removable appliance therapy. Simple intra-maxillary anchorage is most commonly used, anchoring the movement of a few teeth with a larger number of teeth within the same arch (Fig. 13.3). As anchorage is so important for the success of most treatments, movement in removable appliance therapy is usually confined to two teeth at a time so that several other teeth are available for anchorage. If reciprocal anchorage is appropriate, of course, anchorage problems are diminished. Reinforcement of anchorage, where necessary, is also possible with removable appliances. Anchorage reinforcement is most often necessary when teeth are being moved distally, as there is always a greater tendency for anchor teeth to move forward than backward. The decision on whether anchorage reinforcement is necessary depends on two factors:

1 The size and number of the anchor teeth in relation to the moving force.
2 The amount of space available for the tooth movement.

As outlined in Chapter 12, it is necessary, when designing a removable appliance, to ensure that the force on each anchor tooth is less than 0.1 N. This is done by calculating the total force component of the appliance and dividing the sum by the number of anchor teeth. If the result is greater than 0.1 N, it is advisable to reinforce the anchorage to reduce unwanted tooth movement to a minimum. Instruments are available for measuring the force applied by springs and elastics.

The amount of space available for the desired tooth movement must be considered. Simple anchorage is rarely stationary. Even when the force on each anchor tooth is less than 0.1 N there may be slight movement of the anchor teeth. If the space available for the desired tooth movement is only just adequate at the beginning of treatment, even slight movement of the anchor teeth will result in deficiency of space. Therefore, when there is no excess of space it is wise to reinforce anchorage (see Fig. 17.6). This is particularly important in distal movement of teeth, as has been previously mentioned.

For the purpose of distal movement of teeth with removable appliances, anchorage reinforcement can readily be brought about by extra-oral forces. In order to completely stabilize the position of the anchor teeth, the extra-oral force should cancel out the reciprocal action to the force component in the appliance. Since the extra-oral traction is normally worn by the patient for only about 50% of the time, it is necessary to incorporate in it a force at least double that of the force component in the appliance.

When extra-oral traction is used to provide the main force component for tooth movement, the forces necessary must be calculated according to the number of teeth to be moved.

Other methods of reinforcing anchorage with removable appliances, such as the use of inclined bite planes (Fig. 13.2) or the use of arch wires to prevent tipping of anchor teeth, are less precise in their action than extra-oral traction, and the amount of reinforcement provided, in terms of force, cannot be defined. The banding of anchor teeth to prevent tipping can also be used in conjunction with removable appliances. Such an appliance system would fall within the category of fixed—removable combination. Again, the amount of anchorage reinforcement obtained cannot be determined precisely.

Connecting framework

The connecting framework in a removable appliance is usually made from acrylic resin. Its main function is to provide a base for the other components of the appliance, but it does add a little to the retention and anchorage properties. In addition, the framework can be constructed to supply a valuable supplement to the main components of the appliance in the form of *bite planes*. These are areas of the appliance where the framework is built up to prevent normal closure of the mandible, thus preventing normal occlusal contact of the teeth. Three types of bite plane are in common use:

POSTERIOR BITE PLANES

The posterior bite plane consists of capping extending partly or completely across the occlusal surfaces of the buccal teeth (Fig. 13.4). Its purpose is to 'unlock' the occlusion by preventing complete closure of the jaw, so that teeth can be moved across the line of the opposing dental arch. It is most commonly used in appliances to move instanding upper anterior teeth forward, though it is only necessary if there is more than a slight degree of positive incisal overbite. The posterior bite plane should be of sufficient thickness to just overcome the interlocking of the incisor teeth in occlusion. It is also used when moving buccal teeth across the line of the opposing arch.

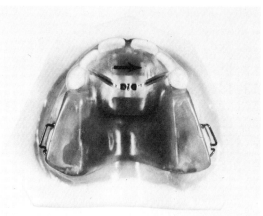

Fig. 13.4. Removable appliance with screw to procline the upper incisors, and posterior bite plane to unlock the occlusion. Anchorage is little problem, since the buccal teeth are resistant to distal movement.

FLAT ANTERIOR BITE PLANES

The flat anterior bite plane is used on upper removable appliances, and is made by building up the base material behind the upper incisors so that the lower anterior teeth touch the bite plane before the buccal teeth come into occlusion (Fig. 13.1). Its main purpose is to reduce the incisal overbite. This is often necessary in treatment of Class 2 occlusal relationship (see Chapter 17) and in certain other conditions. The overbite reduction is probably brought about by continuing vertical development of the lower buccal dento-alveolar structures, which are kept free from occlusal contact by the bite plane (Menezes 1975).

It will be seen from Fig. 13.1 that increased vertical development of the buccal segments will result in an increase in the total vertical dimension of the jaws in occlusion. As this vertical dimension is probably governed by genetically determined neuro-muscular and skeletal growth factors, it seems likely that the artificial increase brought about by the use of the anterior bite plane can only be satisfactorily obtained on a growing child who has not reached full potential dimensions. Provided the artificially increased dimension does not exceed the inherited potential it seems that such a method of reducing incisal overbite is satisfactory. On an adult whose growth is completed, such a method would produce an excessive vertical dimension of the jaws which may interfere with normal function.

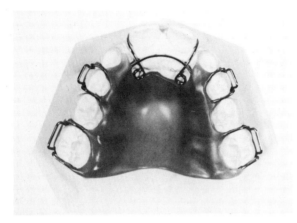

Fig. 13.5. Removable appliance to close an upper median diastema, using reciprocal anchorage.

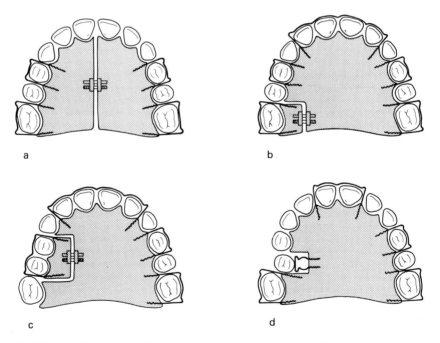

Fig. 13.6. Appliances for the lateral movement of teeth. (a) Simple bilateral expansion using reciprocal anchorage. Molar capping may be necessary to relieve occlusal locking. (b, c) Expansion of separate components of the arch. These appliances used consecutively would tend to produce unilateral expansion. (d) T spring with fixed ends to move a single tooth. The central bends allow the spring to be lengthened.

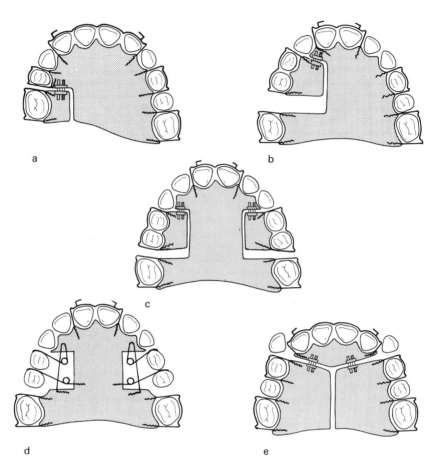

Fig. 13.7. Appliances for the distal movement of buccal teeth. Extra oral anchorage is usually desirable for distal movement of buccal teeth. Screws (in a, b, c, e) should be directed parallel to the line of the arch. Bite planes may be necessary to relieve occlusal locking. To avoid anchorage slip in appliances in (c) and (e) movement on one side should be completed before activating the other side. In appliance (d) only two springs should be active at any time.

INCLINED ANTERIOR BITE PLANES

Inclined anterior bite planes are sometimes used instead of flat bite planes on upper removable appliances. The two types differ only in shape, and both types effect a reduction in incisal overbite. The inclined bite plane can also induce a forward posture of the mandible in Class 2 Division 1 occlusions and thus act as a simple functional appliance (see Chapter 15).

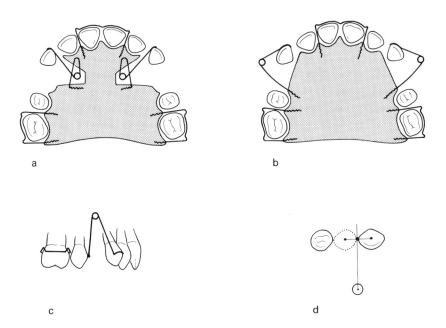

a   b

c   d

Fig. 13.8. Appliances for distal movement of canine teeth. (a) The springs may be open or boxed. Open springs are easier to clean and activate, boxed springs are stronger. (a, b) An anterior bite plane may be necessary for reduction of the overbite. (b, c) The buccal canine retractor is more suitable for outstanding canine teeth with mesial tilt. (d) The coils of the springs should be positioned on a perpendicular to the centre of a line between the old and the new tooth positions. For mesial movement of canine and other teeth the action of the spring can be reversed (see Fig. 13.5).

In general, provided they are carefully designed, with proper attention given to retention, to the degree and quality of the force component, and particularly to the anchorage component, removable appliances can give a valuable contribution to orthodontic treatment. They should not be used to attempt to bring about tooth movements beyond their scope, which is essentially tipping and some simple rotational movement, and the importance of the patient's role in their use must be remembered. On the whole, removable appliances are much more successful in the upper arch than in the lower arch because the shape of the upper jaw facilitates fitting and wearing these appliances. They also interfere less with tongue function in the upper arch.

Types of removable appliance

A large variety of active removable appliances is in common use. Most clinicians have their own favourite appliance designs for various tooth

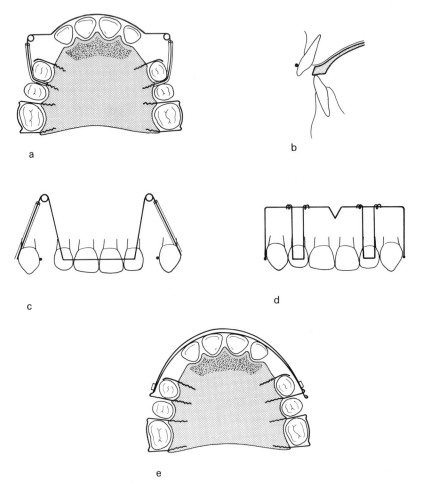

a

b

c

d

e

Fig. 13.9. Appliances for retroclination of incisor teeth. (a, b, c) Roberts' retractor. Maintenance of overbite reduction with anterior bite plane is essential. Trimming of the bite plane is necessary, as shown in (b). (d) A high labial arch with apron spring(s) can be used for retroclination of one or more incisors. (e) Strap spring on labial arch. Bite plane must be trimmed as in (b). Other appliances shown in Figs. 12.2 and 13.3.

movements, and although the range of design is large, it is possible to reduce this range to relatively few designs. The following (Figs. 13.6–13.11) represent a small range of appliances which would carry out most of the movements possible with removable appliances. These are not exclusive, and many variations exist. The one important feature is that the principles of *retention, force application* and *anchorage* must always be observed.

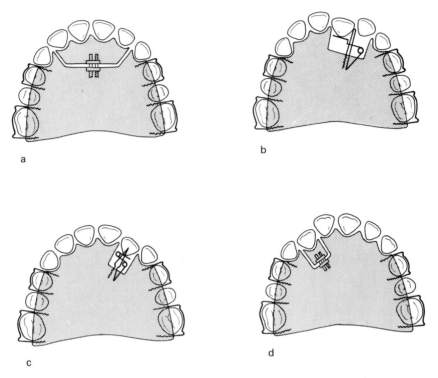

Fig. 13.10. Appliances for proclination of upper incisors. Molar capping may be necessary to relieve occlusal locking. (a) Incisors move more readily if not clasped together. (b) Spring arm may be cranked to give longer range under control of the guard. (c) Z spring may be boxed, or made with extending guard. Multiple Z springs need very good retention. (d) Small screws may be easier than springs for the less skilful patient.

Summary

Removable appliances are limited to tipping and simple rotary movements of teeth, which are sufficient for many orthodontic treatments. They depend on co-operation and a certain degree of skill on the part of the patient.

Components

1 *Retention*—mainly provided by Adams clasps.
2 *Force component*—mainly provided by springs, elastics and screws.
3 *Anchorage component*—usually simple or reciprocal anchorage.
　　Anchorage should be calculated by dividing the total force component by the number of anchor teeth. If more than 0.1 N per anchor

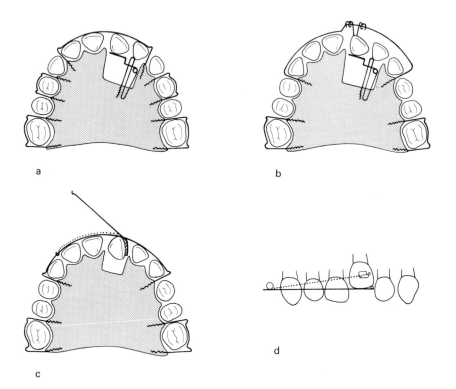

Fig. 13.11. Appliances for simple rotation and vertical movement. (a) A simple palatal spring and labial stop to rotate round the mesial aspect of the incisor. (b) A force couple from a palatal spring and an apron spring to rotate round the centre of the tooth. (c) Whip spring fixed to the tooth via a band or bonded attachment (see also Fig. 14.11). (d) Simple vertical movement needs a fixed attachment on the tooth. Bonded composite resin with a notch gives a seating for a free-ended spring from the removable appliance.

tooth, reinforcement is desirable. Reinforcement is also desirable if there is no excess of space for the tooth movement, particularly with distal movement.

- *Anchorage reinforcement* can be achieved with removable appliances, using extra-oral traction, arch wires or bands, and possibly inclined bite planes.

4 *Connecting framework*, which can be extended to form bite planes.
   - *Posterior bite plane*—for 'unlocking' the occlusion to move teeth across the line of the opposing arch.
   - *Flat anterior bite plane*—for reducing incisal overbite.
   - *Inclined anterior bite plane*—for reducing incisal overbite.

References

Adams, C. P. (1950) The modified arrowhead clasp. *Dent Rec*, **70**, 143–144.

Adams, C. P. (1953) The modified arrowhead clasp—some further considerations. *Dent Rec*, **73**, 332–333.

Adams, C. P. (1984) *The Design and Construction of Removable Orthodontic Appliances*, 5th edn. Bristol, John Wright and Sons Ltd.

Bass, T. P. & Stevens, C. D. (1970) Some experiments with orthodontic springs. *Dent Practit*, **21**, 21–32.

Menezes, D. M. (1975) Changes in the dento-facial complex as a result of bite plane therapy. *Am J Orthod*, **67**, 660–676.

14

Principles of fixed appliance treatment

Fixed appliances form the second major division of orthodontic appliance systems. They have certain important advantages, as well as certain disadvantages, when compared with removable appliances. These may be considered as follows.

Advantages of fixed appliances

1 Retention presents no problem, since the appliance is fixed to the teeth. This means that there is no dislodgement of the appliance by the force component, and multiple forces can be applied to the teeth simultaneously, thus facilitating multiple tooth movement and, in some circumstances, reducing the time required for treatment.
2 Less skill is required from the patient in management of the appliance. Again, this facilitates multiple simultaneous tooth movement which would be difficult with a removable appliance without complicating the appliance beyond the patient's capabilities.
3 It is possible to bring about tooth movements with fixed appliances which are not possible with removable appliances. This is because, by and large, removable appliances apply their force component only to a very small area of the crown of the tooth, and can therefore produce only tipping and simple rotational movements. As will be seen later, it is possible with fixed appliances to apply the force component over a wider area of the crown of the tooth, and to control movement so that bodily and torquing movements are produced. This is the main advantage of fixed appliance treatment, and the main reason for its use.

Fixed appliances are thus not to be regarded as an alternative to removable appliances, but provide an extra dimension in orthodontic treatment, considerably expanding its scope in some of the more complex occlusal problems.

Disadvantages of fixed appliances

The main potential disadvantage centres round the problem of oral health. Appliances fixed to the teeth are more difficult to clean than removable appliances, and it is more difficult to maintain oral health during appliance treatment. With care, and a well-motivated and capable patient, this problem can be avoided.

A further potential disadvantage is the possibility of producing adverse tooth movement. With the appliance fixed to the teeth, excessive force will not cause dislodgement and may therefore damage the supporting structures of the teeth. Furthermore, in the more complex fixed appliance systems it is easy to achieve unwanted movement through reciprocal forces, and these systems should only be applied by experienced operators.

Components of fixed appliances

Fixed appliances act through attachments fitted directly to the teeth. The attachments may be welded to stainless steel bands which are cemented to the teeth, or may be bonded to the teeth through one of the acid-etch retained bonding systems. Several different systems of bonding are in use, using either mechanical retention to metal mesh or ceramic attachments or chemical retention to plastic attachments. Many of the systems have been compared and evaluated (Delport & Grobler 1988; Gwinnett 1988), but the bonding of attachments is still in an early stage of development and it is likely that there will be continuous changes and improvements.

The attachments broadly consist of tubes, brackets and hooks to which the force component can be fitted. There is such a wide variety of types of attachment that only a brief general description can be given here.

Tubes, which are usually fitted to the last molars in the arch, may be round or rectangular in section, to take either round or rectangular section archwire. Larger tubes are used to take extra-oral arches.

Brackets are usually fitted to all other anchor teeth and teeth which are to be moved. There are two main types of bracket, with many modifications. The edgewise bracket has a rectangular-section slot into which the archwire fits, and spurs for tying in the archwire with some form of ligature. The bracket is made in a variety of widths and sometimes double or treble brackets are fitted. The slots may also be angulated and this is the basis of the straight wire system devised by Andrews (1976). With the edgewise bracket the width of the attachment is important, since it gives control over the tooth movement in a mesio-distal dimension. Furthermore, the rectangular slot, when used in conjunction with an archwire of rectangular section, gives control over tooth movement in a labio-lingual or bucco-lingual dimension, because the archwire cannot rotate in the slot (Fig. 14.1).

The Begg bracket (Fig. 14.2) differs in that effectively it has no width

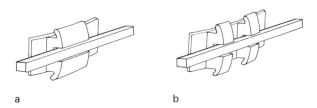

a   b

Fig. 14.1. The basic edgewise bracket. (a) Single bracket; and (b) double bracket. Archwire of rectangular section fits accurately in the bracket slot and can produce movement in a mesio-distal or bucco-lingual direction.

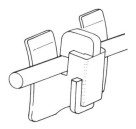

Fig. 14.2. The Begg bracket. In this light wire bracket the archwire is pinned relatively loosely in the bracket slot and the tooth can tip or rotate freely on the archwire.

and no precise location of the archwire, so that the teeth can tip or rotate freely under the influence of the force component. It is almost always used with archwire of round section, and the force component is either built into the archwire or added in the form of auxiliary springs. The archwire is held loosely in the bracket by means of a soft metal pin.

Hooks, buttons and cleats can also be added to the teeth for attachment of auxiliary forces.

The force component usually consists of stainless steel springs or arches, or elastics (Figs. 14.3–14.5). Fairly precise regulation of the forces can be achieved, but, as mentioned above the reciprocal forces need to be carefully controlled.

The anchorage component can be achieved from simple anchorage or reciprocal anchorage. Intermaxillary traction is commonly used in some fixed appliance systems, and is much more successful than with removable appliances, where the retention problems tend to make intermaxillary traction unsatisfactory. Anchorage reinforcement with extra-oral traction is also commonly used in fixed appliance treatment.

Principles of anchorage are, of course, the same as for removable appliances, but some small differences are possible in methods of achieving anchorage. Some or all of the anchor teeth are almost in-

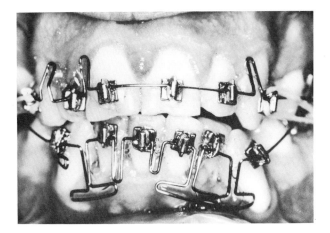

Fig. 14.3. Fixed appliance using the distortion of an archwire to move the teeth. The loops in the wire increase its length and flexibility.

variably banded, and are thus more resistant to tipping. Therefore, if the active tooth movement to be achieved is only a tipping movement, anchorage with fixed appliances is usually good, provided sufficient anchor teeth are available. If, on the other hand, bodily or torquing movements are to be achieved, anchorage may become more difficult because of the extra forces needed for these movements. In some systems the anchor teeth are deliberately tipped in the opposite direction to the reciprocal force before active tooth movement is started, so that they will provide extra anchorage.

Types of fixed appliances

Any orthodontic appliance which is fixed to the teeth comes under the general description of 'fixed appliance'. There are, however, many different fixed appliance systems in use, which vary considerably in their methods of achieving tooth movement and in the details of their component parts. Certain principles of treatment run through these various systems, and these can be examined by a review of a few of the types of appliance available.

THE LABIO-LINGUAL SYSTEM

Labio-lingual appliances consist essentially of bands on the anchor teeth, usually the first permanent molars, and a labial, lingual or palatal

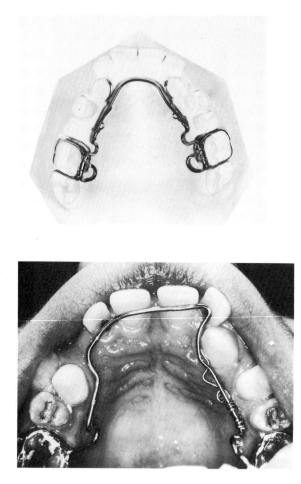

Fig. 14.4. The labio-lingual system. Lingual arches with springs to move upper canine teeth. Only the anchor and retention teeth are banded, and the moving teeth can only be tilted.

arch attached to the bands. The arch is used for the application of force to the teeth to be moved, which are not themselves banded. The force can be applied by means of springs attached to the arch (Fig. 14.4) or by elastics. It is possible with this system to apply intermaxillary or extra-oral traction.

It will be seen that, since the moving teeth are not banded, the force can only be applied over a small area of the crown. This is exactly the same as with removable appliances, and, on the whole, only tipping movements or simple rotations can be achieved. The labio-lingual system has certain advantages over removable appliances. Anchorage

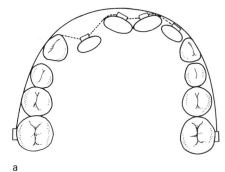

a

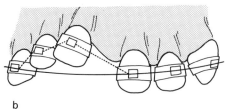

b

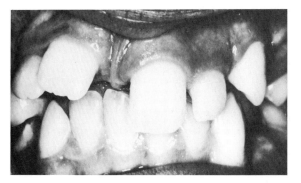

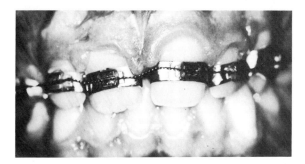

Fig. 14.5. Tooth movement with multiband appliance (1). The flexible archwire is formed to an ideal arch form in its passive position. (b) When distorted and attached to the misplaced teeth, it returns towards the passive position, bringing the teeth with it.

may be better, since the anchor teeth are banded. Retention of the appliance is obviously better. Patient skills are not needed, apart from oral hygiene. On the whole, however, the labio-ligual system does not bring much to orthodontic treatment that removable appliances cannot provide.

MULTIBAND OR MULTIBOND APPLIANCE SYSTEMS

The attachment of components to the teeth which are to be moved brings the appliance within the category of multiband or multibond systems, and adds a new dimension to treatment. A much wider range of tooth movements becomes possible, and, in theory at least, the precise control of tooth position is limited only by the skeletal and oromuscular environment and the skill and knowledge of the operator. The force component is applied over a wide area of the tooth and it is relatively easy to apply force couples and restricting forces.

Two general principles of achieving tooth movement can be outlined, though there is considerable overlap between the two.

1   The distortion of a flexible arch from its passive position (Fig. 14.5)

A resilient flexible archwire will tend to return to its passive position when distorted. If such an archwire is formed so that its passive position corresponds to the position into which it is desired to move the teeth, it can be distorted and attached to the teeth which are to be moved, and in returning to its passive position it will apply force to the teeth in the required direction.

This principle underlies much of multiband appliance treatment, and it can be seen from Fig. 14.5 that it can produce movement in all planes of space. The position of the anchor teeth should correspond to the passive position of the archwire unless reciprocal movement is required. It is not necessary for a complete archwire to be used. A partial arch, corresponding essentially to a spring, can be used to work on the same principle (Fig. 14.6).

2   The use of passive archwire as a guide

A passive archwire attached to the anchor teeth and to the teeth to be moved can be used to guide and control movement. In this case the force component is added, usually by means of an elastic or a helical coiled spring (Fig. 14.7).

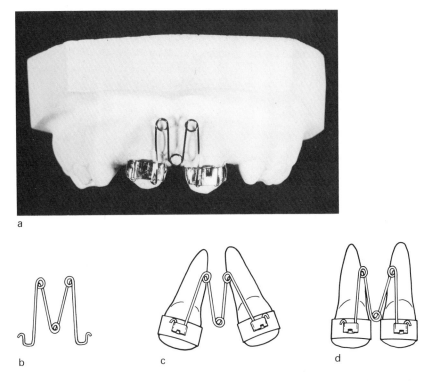

Fig. 14.6. (a) Model with M spring in position. (b) M spring in passive position. (c) Spring activated and attached to displaced teeth. (d) Spring returned to passive position, moving apices and crowns of the teeth.

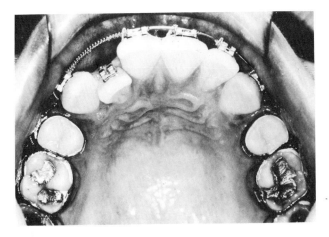

Fig. 14.7. Tooth movement with multiband appliance (2). Coil spring to produce distal movement of the upper canine tooth, the archwire acting as a guide.

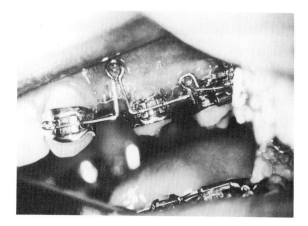

Fig. 14.8. Sectional multiband appliance to retract an upper canine tooth.

All multiband appliances function by means of these principles, many appliance systems using both, often simultaneously.

SECTIONAL MULTIBAND APPLIANCES

It is not always necessary to fit a multiband appliance to the whole dental arch. Sometimes, for localized tooth movements, it is sufficient to fit attachments only on one segment of the arch. Such appliances are known as *sectional appliances,* and they are useful for producing tooth movements which could not be achieved with removable appliances, but which do not need the complexity of a full multiband system (Fig. 14.8).

Tooth movements with multiband appliances

There are many ways of producing the various types of tooth movement with multiband appliances. A few of these methods will be outlined to illustrate some appliances in common use.

TIPPING MOVEMENTS

Tipping movements are the most easily produced by any appliance system. Multiband appliances to produce such movements are illustrated in Figs. 14.3 and 14.9.

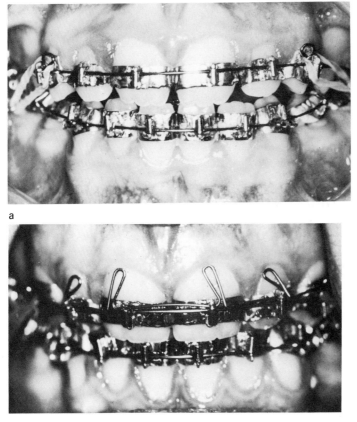

a

b

Fig. 14.9. Bodily movement by tipping followed by apical torque. (a) Intermaxillary elastics tip back the upper incisors. (b) The spurs on the archwire produce a force couple for apical torque.

ROTATIONAL MOVEMENTS

Rotations are usually brought about by utilizing the flexibility and resilience of the archwire. The flexibility can be increased by incorporating more wire in the arch in the form of loops or coils (see Fig. 14.3). Rotations can also be achieved by adding extra forces in the form of elastic ligatures.

BODILY MOVEMENTS

True bodily movement, without tilting, can only be accomplished with rigid control over the tooth. It is best accomplished using an archwire of

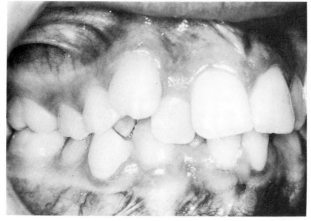

a

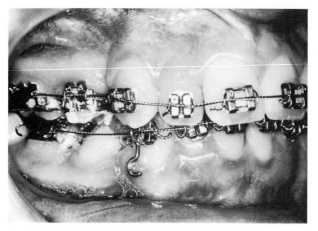

b

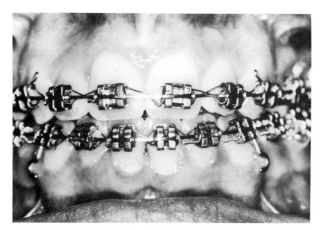

c

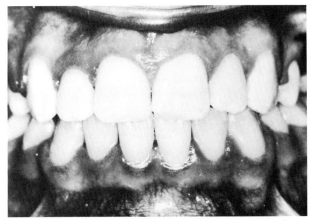

d

Fig. 14.10. A variety of tooth movements in the treatment of a Class 2 occlusion with crowding. (a) The original condition. The first premolars are to be extracted. (b) A flexible multistrand arch correcting the main irregularities. (c) A rectangular arch engaged in the angulated bracket slots, effecting overbite reduction and arch alignment and allowing bodily retraction of the upper incisors via intermaxillary traction. (d) The final position of the incisor teeth.

rectangular section which fits accurately in a bracket of the same shape and size. Unwanted movements are thus avoided, tooth position being accurately governed by the position of the archwire. This is the basis of the edgewise appliance system. As greater force is required to move teeth bodily, the force on the anchor teeth is greater than for any other movement, and anchorage must be carefully planned. A sectional appliance producing bodily movement is illustrated in Fig. 14.8.

The effect of bodily movement can also be achieved in another way, by first tipping the tooth and then uprighting it with apical torque, using a secondary force to prevent crown movement (Fig. 14.9).

TORQUING MOVEMENTS

Root torque is produced by applying force to the crown of the tooth and restricting crown movement. It can only be done satisfactorily with multiband appliances. It can be achieved with archwires and brackets of rectangular section or by applying a force couple, using loops to apply force to two points on the tooth with the same archwire, the latter being a stage in the Begg appliance system (Fig. 14.9). In both cases crown movement is restricted by tying back the archwire or a secondary archwire to the anchor teeth.

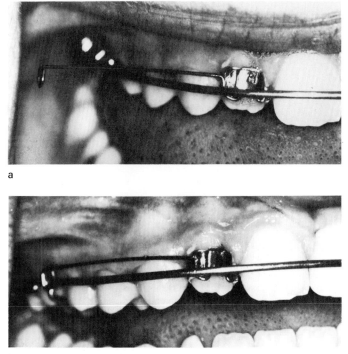

a

b

Fig. 14.11. Fixed–removable combination appliance. Whip spring to rotate a tooth.
(a) The spring in its passive position attached to the tooth. (b) The spring activated and
hooked to the archwire of a removable appliance, producing a rotary force. The archwire
also acts as a stop to prevent the tooth moving forward.

VERTICAL MOVEMENTS

Extrusion and intrusion of teeth are possible with multiband systems,
using the flexibility of an archwire to apply the appropriate forces (see
Fig. 14.5b).

Fig. 14.10 shows a variety of movements applied in the treatment of
a Class 2 occlusion with crowding.

Fixed–removable appliance combinations

It is sometimes of value to combine the properties of fixed and
removable appliances to achieve the advantages of both. Generally
speaking, such combined appliances are used for localized tooth
movements of a type which could not be achieved with removable

appliances alone, but the use of a removable component facilitates oral hygiene and makes the construction of the appliance more simple. An example of this type of appliance is shown in Fig. 14.11.

It should be remembered that fixed appliances, particularly multi-band systems, are capable of applying considerable forces to the teeth. Reciprocal forces can also readily produce adverse tooth movement. The purpose of this chapter has been to outline the principles behind their use. Successful practice in their use requires training and experience.

References

Andrews, L. F. (1976) The straight wire appliance explained and compared. *J Clin Orthod*, **12**, 569–586.

Delport, A. & Grobler, S. R. (1988) A laboratory evaluation of the tensile bond strength of some orthodontic resins to enamel. *Am J Orthod*, **93**, 133–137.

Gwinnett, A. J. (1988) A comparison of shear bond strengths of metal and ceramic brackets. *Am J Orthod*, **93**, 346–348.

15

Principles of functional appliance treatment

Functional appliances are mostly removable appliances, but are considered separately here because the force component in a functional appliance is quite different from that in any other type of removable appliance. Whereas the active removable appliances, described in Chapter 13, derive their force component from springs, screws or elastics, the force components in functional appliances originate in the oro-facial and masticatory musculature.

Functional appliances have been, and still are, the subject of a certain amount of controversy regarding their mode of action. It is generally accepted that they produce tooth movement by applying force directly to the teeth. In addition, it is claimed that some appliances can induce bone growth which will enlarge the basal parts of the jaws and bring about favourable changes in the dental base relationships, thus helping to correct crowding and discrepancies in dental arch relationships. It is these latter claims regarding bone growth which have been disputed by many authorities.

The mode of action of functional appliances

Several types of functional appliance have been introduced. Although they differ in detail, their action falls into three categories.
1 Utilizing the forces of the muscles of mastication.
2 Utilizing the forces of the circumoral musculature.
3 Reducing the forces of the circumoral musculature.

Almost all functional appliances use the principles embodied in two basic appliances, the Andresen appliance or activator, and the oral or vestibular screen. Many appliances combine the principles of these two basic appliances.

The Andresen appliance

The Andresen appliance, activator or monobloc consists of a single block of base material into which both upper and lower dental arches fit (Fig. 15.1). Archwires are incorporated to apply appropriate forces to the teeth. It is most frequently used in the correction of Class 2 dental arch relationship. The essence of the appliance is that it is made so that it fits

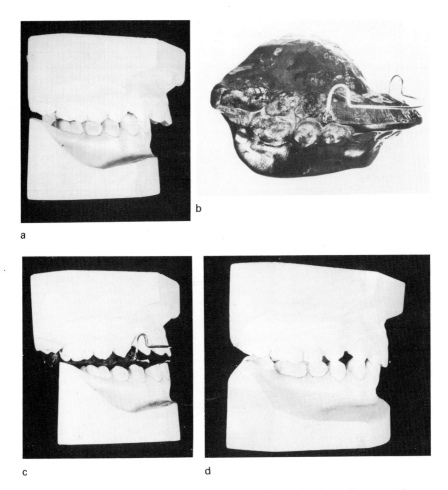

Fig. 15.1. The Andresen appliance. (a) Models in occlusion. (b) The appliance. (c) The mandible is postured forward to fit the appliance. (d) Final models.

the upper arch, and the lower arch will only fit into the appliance with the mandible in a predetermined postured position. Thus, when it is worn the muscles of mastication are stretched beyond their position of postural tonus. It has been suggested that this has two effects.

1 The muscles of mastication exert a force on the mandible in attempting to return to their resting position. This results in a force being exerted on the mandibular teeth and an opposite force on the maxillary teeth via the appliance, i.e. a form of intermaxillary traction.

2 The postural position of the mandible modifies or induces growth at

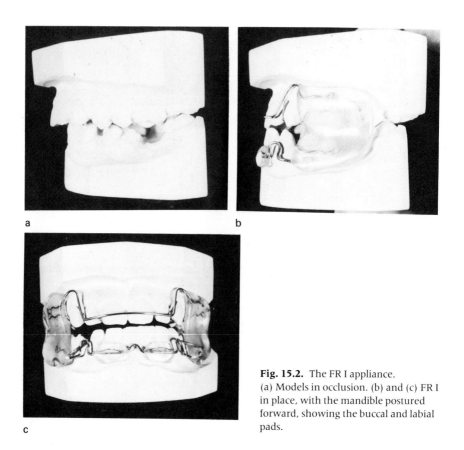

Fig. 15.2. The FR I appliance.
(a) Models in occlusion. (b) and (c) FR I
in place, with the mandible postured
forward, showing the buccal and labial
pads.

the mandibular condyles and temporo-mandibular joint fossae, which effectively alters the basal bone relationship.

The first of these effects probably does occur, and is responsible for tooth movement through the alveolar bone. With regard to the second effect, a good deal of evidence has been presented in attempts to show that bone growth is induced, but this is far from being universally accepted at present. Further consideration of this point will be made at the end of the chapter.

Apart from the application of the main forces to the upper teeth via the labial arch and the lower teeth via the lingual base material, it is usual to trim the Andresen appliance to facilitate tooth movement. The appliance is trimmed behind the upper incisors so that they may tilt palatally, and between the upper and lower buccal teeth so that the upper teeth may move distally and the lower teeth mesially. The trimming is usually made to allow occlusal movement of the buccal teeth,

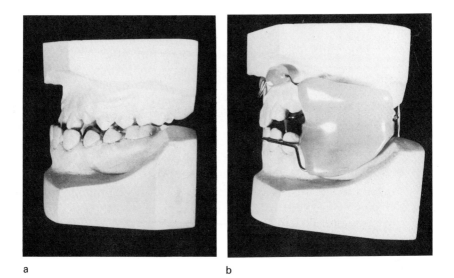

a   b

Fig. 15.3. The FR III appliance. (a) Models in occlusion. (b) FR III in place with incisor teeth edge-to-edge, showing the labial pad.

but the lower incisors are prevented from moving occlusally if excessive incisal overbite needs correction.

Owing to its bulky nature, the Andresen appliance is not normally worn during daytime, since it would interfere with speaking, eating and respiration during physical exertion. Like any other part-time appliance, it has the disadvantage that it applies intermittent forces to the teeth. In practice, this is not normally a problem except when there is a severe lip-trap, the lower lip putting a forward force on the upper incisors during the day which counteracts the force of the appliance at night. In such circumstances the Andresen appliance is not usually the best choice for treatment.

The oral or vestibular screen

This appliance, on its own, has very limited application and is not often used, but the principle of its use is incorporated in several other types of functional appliance. As the name implies, it is a screen of base material which is made to fit in the vestibule of the mouth. By differential relief of various areas on the construction models it can be used either to apply the forces of the circumoral musculature to certain teeth, or to relieve those forces from the teeth, thus producing or allowing tooth movement. As a full screen it can only be worn part-time, since it interferes with other oral functions. However, as a partial screen, in which form the principle is frequently used in other appliances, it can often be worn for much of the time apart from when eating.

Other functional appliances

All other functional appliances use the two forementioned principles. Most appliance systems emphasize one particular aspect of functional treatment, and this is perhaps the reason for the multiplicity of functional appliance systems which exist at present.

The Fränkel function corrector

The Fränkel appliance embodies the principles of both the Andresen appliance and the oral screen. It is made to a postured occlusion to utilize the forces of the masticatory muscles and it carries screens to relieve the forces of the circumoral musculature.

Two basic appliances are described (Fränkel 1980), the Function Corrector I (FR I) for the treatment of Class 1 and Class 2 Division 1 occlusions, and the Function Corrector III (FR III) for the treatment of Class 3 occlusions.

The FR I consists of a wire framework comprising a palatal bar, a lower lingual arch and an upper labial arch. Attached to the wire frame is a buccal pad on each side and two labial pads (Fig. 15.2). These pads fit in the vestibule of the mouth, and their function is to hold the cheeks and lower lip away from the teeth. For the correction of Class 2 relationship the whole appliance is made to fit the jaws with the mandible in a forward postural position.

The FR III is similar except that its action is reversed. The lingual arch is behind the upper incisors and the labial arch is in front of the lower incisors. The labial pads lie in the upper labial sulcus, and hold the upper lip away from the teeth (Fig. 15.3). The appliance is made to fit the mandible in a retruded position (Eirew *et al.* 1976).

After an initial introductory period, the Fränkel appliance is worn full-time except when eating, as in most patients it does not interfere severely with oral function.

Thus, in use in the treatment of Class 2 and Class 3 occlusions, the Fränkel appliance can apply force to the teeth from the muscles of mastication. It is also claimed that it acts in three other ways.

1 The forward postural position induces growth at the mandibular condyle and temporo-mandibular joint.

2 The vestibular pads, by preventing adverse muscle pressures on the teeth, induce growth of the basal bone of the jaws, thus allowing enlargement of the dental arches and relief of crowding.

3 The labial vestibular pads, by altering muscle position and action, induce favourable growth of the lips.

Many other functional appliances have been designed.

The *Propulsor* (Hotz 1974) is a combination of a monobloc activator and partial oral screen, usually without any wire components.

The *Kinetor* (Stockfisch 1971) is an activator with wire buccal shields which may incorporate screws and springs to produce forces independent of the functional muscular component.

The *Bimler appliance* (Bimler 1973) is an activator largely made from wire components, with differential screening of the cheeks and lips, and with the possibility of incorporating screws for arch expansion.

The *Bionator* (Eirew 1981) is a largely wire-based activator with wire buccal screens and acrylic base material to locate the mandible in a postured occlusal position. In one form it incorporates a lingual screen to prevent abnormal tongue activity.

The *Harvold activator* (Harvold & Vargervik 1971; Reed & Hathorn 1978) has similarities to the Andresen appliance in that it is essentially an acrylic monobloc which is made to a postured mandibular position, but it differs in important respects. It is made to a mandibular position opened beyond the resting position in order to harness the forces of the stretched circumoral and facial tissues, and certain inter-occlusal sections of the appliance are omitted to allow differential dento-alveolar development.

The *Clark twin-block* (Clark 1988) consists of separate upper and lower removable appliances, each with a 45° posterior bite plane designed to induce a mandibular posture of the desired amount and direction. One or both sections may incorporate a mid-line screw to effect arch expansion, and there is provision for the addition of extra-oral traction.

The effects of functional appliance treatment

There is little doubt that functional appliances produce tooth movement and in many cases can correct occlusal discrepancies. The controversy over their use relates mainly to their mode of action, and in particular to two aspects. The first is the question of modification of growth of the basal parts of the jaws. Many authorities believe that basal jaw growth can be altered by functional means. The temporo-mandibular joint area has been thought to be a reactive growth site, i.e. any prolonged change in the position of the mandible during the growth period, such as is induced by wearing the appliance, results in bone apposition on the mandibular and temporal surfaces of the enlarged joint cavity. Baume (1969) quotes histological evidence to support this concept, and ample clinical evidence has been produced in attempts to show that the use of functional appliances can alter the skeletal relationship of the jaws. For example, Birkebaek *et al.* (1984) studied the effects of the Harvold appliance in Class 2 occlusions, and concluded that they produced an increase in the amount and a change in the direction of mandibular growth together with remodelling of the articular fossae. Both Dugger (1982) and Haynes (1986) have found that the Fränkel appliance produced an increase in mandibular length when used in treatment of Class 2 occlusions. On the other hand, this clinical evidence does not always take into account the effects of normal growth. As functional appliances are normally used during the mixed dentition stage a considerable amount of normal growth must occur which could alter jaw size and relationships. Several investigators have failed to find evidence of altered growth with functional appliances, but instead have found the main effects to be tipping of the incisors and an opening rotation of the mandible (Calvert 1982; Mörndal, 1984; Loh & Kerr, 1985; Hamilton *et al.* 1987). Cohen (1981), in a study of Class 2 Division 1 cases treated by the Andresen appliance, found that those showing the more complete overjet reduction also showed more and faster growth in facial height.

With regard to the effects of relieving muscle pressures on the teeth with the use of buccal and labial pads, Fränkel (1980) feels that these pressures are abnormal in many patients with malocclusion, and that they restrict growth. The advocates of functional appliance therapy claim that the removal of these abnormal pressures enhances unrestricted growth up to the patient's inherent potential, tending to relieve dental arch crowding and discrepancies in arch relationship. Increases in the width of the dental arches have been demonstrated by Dugger (1982), Brieden *et al.* (1984) and Hamilton *et al.* (1987) among others, though such increases are not necessarily enough to relieve severe crowding.

Thus the differences of opinion regarding the action of functional appliances are still unresolved. Without doubt, they can produce changes in the position of the teeth, and in suitable circumstances they provide a valuable method of orthodontic treatment. It may be that the apparent effects on bone growth which they sometimes seem to induce could be the result of individual variation in growth rates, the more favourable effects occurring during periods when growth would readily bring changes.

Summary

Functional appliances provide a valuable method of orthodontic treatment in certain circumstances. They work best in the mixed dentition and during active growth phases. They are claimed to act by:

1 Using forces of the muscles of mastication.
2 Using forces of the oro-facial muscles.
3 Inducing tooth movement and bone growth by relieving adverse muscle forces on the dentition.
4 Inducing change in the basal part of the jaws, by modifying mandibular or maxillary growth.

Functional appliances incorporate two principles:

1 The 'activator' principle of a forced mandibular posture, which places intermaxillary forces on the teeth and jaws via the masticatory and facial muscles.
2 The 'screening' principle, which harnesses or relieves direct forces on the teeth from the circumoral muscles.

Though the direct forces on the teeth cause tooth movement, there is not general agreement that functional appliances can modify basal bone growth. There is evidence to suggest that temporo-mandibular growth is reactive, but bone growth concomitant with the use of functional appliances may be no more than normal growth processes.

References

Baume, L. J. (1969) Cephalo-facial growth patterns and the functional adaptation of the temporo-mandibular joint structures. *Eur Orthod Soc Trans*, pp. 79–98.

Bimler, H. P. (1973) Dynamic functional therapy. The Bimler appliance. *Eur Orthod Soc Trans*, pp. 451–456.

Birkebaek, L., Melsen, B. & Terp, S. (1984) A laminagraphic study of the alterations in the temporo-mandibular joint following activator treatment. *Eur J Orthod*, **6**, 257–266.

Brieden, C. M., Pangrazio-Kulbersh, V. & Kulbersh, R. (1984) Maxillary skeletal and dental change with Fränkel appliance therapy—an implant study. *Angle Orthod*, **54**, 226–232.

Calvert, F. J. (1982) An assessment of Andresen therapy on Class II Division I malocclusion. *Br J Orthod*, **9**, 149–153.

Clark, W. J. (1988) The twin-block technique: a functional orthopaedic appliance system. *Am J Orthod*, **93**, 1–18.

Cohen, A. M. (1981) A study of Class 2 Division 1 malocclusions treated by the Andresen appliance. *Br J Orthod*, **8**, 159–163.

Dugger, G. C. (1982) Orofacial change resulting from Fränkel appliance treatment. *Am J Orthod*, **82**, 354 (abstract).

Eirew, H. L. (1981) The Bionator. *Br J Orthod*, **8**, 33–36.

Eirew, H. L., McDowell, F. & Phillips, J. G. (1976). The function regulator of Fränkel. *Br J Orthod*, **3**, 67–74.

Fränkel, R. (1980) A functional approach to orofacial orthopaedics. *Br J Orthod*, **7**, 41–51.

Hamilton, S. D., Sinclair, P. M. & Hamilton, R. H. (1987) A cephalometric, tomographic and dental cast evaluation of Fränkel therapy. *Am J Orthod*, **92**, 427–434.

Harvold, E. P. & Vargervik, K. (1971) Morphogenetic response to activator treatment. *Am J Orthod*, **60**, 478–490.

Haynes, S. (1986) A cephalometric study of mandibular changes in modified function regulator (Fränkel) treatment. *Am J Orthod*, **90**, 308–320.

Hotz, R. P. (1974) *Orthodontics in Daily Practice.* 1st edn. Baltimore, Williams and Wilkins.

Loh, M. K. & Kerr, W. J. S. (1985) The Function Regulator III: effects and indications for use. *Br J Orthod*, **12**, 153–157.

Mörndal, O. (1984) The effect on the incisor teeth of activator treatment: a follow-up study. *Br J Orthod*, **11**, 214–220.

Reed, R. T. & Hathorn, I. S. (1978) The activator. *Br J Orthod*, **5**, 75–80.

Stockfisch, H. (1971) Possibilities and limitations of the Kinetor bimaxillary appliance. *Eur Orthod Soc Trans*, pp. 317–328.

16

Principles of treatment in Class 1 occlusal relationship

In Class 1 occlusions, the antero-posterior relationship of the dental arches is correct. Nevertheless a wide variety of occlusal discrepancies can exist. The most frequent of these are:

- Crowding and irregularity of the teeth.
- Crossbites.
- Excessive overbite.
- Anterior open bite.
- Localized malpositions.

Most of these conditions have been considered in other sections of this book. They are obviously not confined to Class 1 occlusions, but can be seen in any occlusal relationship.

Crowding and irregularity of the teeth

This has been discussed in Chapter 6. It is usually necessary to relieve crowding by extraction of teeth (see Chapter 11) and in Class 1 relationships the extractions usually need to be symmetrical, the objective being to finish with the same number of teeth in each quadrant of the arches. This usually means extractions on each side of both upper and lower arches, though not necessarily of the same teeth in each quadrant.

The simple irregularities of the upper arch can be treated with removable appliances such as those shown in Chapter 13. Malposition of teeth requiring apical or bodily movement needs to be carried out with fixed appliances (see Chapter 14).

The treatment of lower arch crowding in Class 1 occlusion needs special mention since removable appliances are generally less satisfactory in the lower arch. Three aspects can be considered:

1 The site of the crowding.
2 The degree of crowding.
3 The position of individual teeth.

The site of the crowding may be confined to the incisor region, the canines, the premolar or the third molars, or may be a combination of two or more of these sites. Crowding confined to one site is often easier to correct simply by extractions, particularly when confined to premolar or third molar regions.

It is unusual for the total degree of crowding to exceed one premolar unit width in each quadrant.

Extraction of teeth in very mild crowding may result in residual spacing of the arches unless fixed appliances can be used for tooth movement. In more severe crowding, spontaneous space closure may be beneficial but may not allow relief of irregularity without the use of active or passive appliances. Whether adequate spontaneous movment occurs will depend on the position of individual teeth, particularly their apical position and rotations.

In most cases of lower arch crowding the first premolars are chosen for extraction (see Chapter 11). The treatment after such extractions can be summarized as follows:

1   Crowding confined to premolar regions usually needs either no further treatment or simple space maintenance.

2   Crowding of canines: if crowding does not exceed one third of the width of the canine, and the canine apex is in the correct position, spontaneous improvement is likely. If crowding is greater, space maintenance is needed. If the apical position is incorrect, active appliance treatment may be necessary.

3   Crowding of incisors: similar considerations to above. For complete spontaneous alignment the total crowding should not exceed one third of a unit width in each quadrant, otherwise space maintenance or active treatment will be necessary.

The presence of occlusal interlocking on lower canines or incisors will tend to prevent spontaneous movement after extractions. Berg and Gebauer (1982) have found an average spontaneous reduction of about 50% of lower first premolar extraction spaces, with considerable individual variation. Most of the space reduction resulted from distal drifting of lower canines. In the more severe crowding, however, there is a distinct risk of space loss from forward movement of lower second premolars and molars. Stephens (1983) has found that space closure following the extraction of lower first premolars is most rapid in the period immediately following the extraction with little change after the first 3 months.

Crossbites of the buccal teeth have been discussed in Chapter 7. Unilateral crossbite associated with a lateral deviation of mandibular closure should be treated by simple bilateral expansion of the upper dental arch. Bilateral crossbite is often acceptable if it is symmetrical. Treatment usually needs rapid maxillary expansion with fixed appliances to open the mid-palatal suture rather than simply tilt the upper teeth buccally.

Excessive overbite needs correction if it is producing gingival trauma. While the overbite can be reduced by using simple anterior bite planes, a permanent reduction usually requires modification of the incisor angulations to achieve correct interincisal contacts (see Chapter 17). In Class 1 relationship this usually needs fixed appliances to produce torquing movements. Similarly, anterior open bite requires vertical movement of incisor teeth which can only be achieved with the use of fixed appliances.

Other localized malpositions of teeth may be corrected with simple appliances such as shown in Chapter 13, or may need fixed appliances, particularly if several teeth are involved or the apices are malpositioned.

References

Berg, R. & Gebauer, U. (1982) Spontaneous changes in the mandibular arch following first premolar extractions. *Eur J Orthod*, **4**, 93–98.

Stephens, C. D. (1983) The rate of spontaneous closure at the site of extracted mandibular first premolars. *Br J Orthod*, **10**, 93–97.

17

Principles of treatment in Class 2 occlusal relationship

The Class 2 occlusal relationship, in its two main forms, provides the major load of orthodontic appliance treatment in many communities. Foster and Day (1974) have estimated that over 60% of orthodontic appliance treatment in a British community would be involved in treating Class 2 Division 1 or Division 2 occlusions.

Class 2 treatment differs from treatment in Class 1 in having the added complication of antero-posterior dental arch discrepancy. Therefore, in addition to the possible necessity of correcting crowding and irregularity of the teeth and any local anomalies, one of the main objectives in Class 2 treatments is usually the correction of the antero-posterior dental arch relationship.

The two main types of Class 2 relationship have in common the antero-posterior arch discrepancy. Otherwise they show different features, needing rather different treatment, and they will therefore be considered separately.

Class 2 Division 1 occlusion

It is important to appreciate that Class 2 Division 1, as with all other occlusal anomalies, has a wide range of severity in its manifestation, and in its aetiological features. The main variants in the occlusion are, (Figs. 17.1, 17.2, 17.3):

1 The degree of Class 2 discrepancy.
2 The inclination of the incisors and the degree of incisal overjet.
3 The degree of incisal overbite (Fig. 17.2).
4 The degree of crowding of the teeth (Fig. 17.3).

Variation in these features is brought about by variation in the aetiological factors, the main ones being the following.

1 The skeletal relationship is largely responsible for the degree of antero-posterior discrepancy.

2 The form and function, in association with the skeletal relationship, of the muscles of the lips and tongue, govern the inclination and degree of vertical development of the incisors, and thus govern the incisal overjet and overbite.

3 The size of the dentition and of the jaws, which governs the degree of crowding.

It is essential to make a careful assessment of all these features before making a plan for treatment, since some of them impose severe limitations on treatment and the occlusal condition can range from one which is readily corrected by simple measures to one which cannot be fully corrected by orthodontic treatment techniques.

The skeletal relationship may vary from a Class 1 to a severe Class 2 relationship. In the former, the Class 2 Division 1 occlusion is likely to be largely due to muscular factors. In the latter, skeletal and muscular factors will be involved, and will reduce the possibility of full corrective treatment. Indeed, the greater the degree of Class 2 skeletal discrepancy, the more difficult full corrective treatment becomes.

The shape of the lower jaw, particularly at the gonial angle, may also cause variation in the vertical relationship of the upper and lower incisors. A very high gonial angle may be associated with an anterior open bite, which is sometimes beyond correction (Fig. 17.1c). In the opposite situation, a low gonial angle may be associated with a deep incisal overbite (Fig. 17.1a). The difficulty of correction of the latter depends to a large extent on the degree of antero-posterior skeletal discrepancy.

The relative widths of the jaws may vary, and if a severe discrepancy exists between the width of upper and lower jaws, this adds to the severity of the malocclusion and to the difficulty of treatment (Fig. 17.4).

The muscle form and function can show variations even more complex than those of the skeletal factors. To a large extent, the effect of the muscle factors are dependent on the skeletal factors, the muscles being attached to the jaws. Thus an antero-posterior Class 2 skeletal discrepancy will result in the lower lip and tongue being retropositioned in relation to the upper lip and dento-alveolar structures.

The vertical relationship of the lips varies independently of the skeletal relationship. Ideally, the lips have sufficient vertical dimension to be able to meet in the rest position. At the other extreme the lips may be widely apart at rest, and the resultant muscular contraction necessary for lip closure may have a marked effect on the inclination of the incisor teeth, particularly the lower incisors. Many individuals with Class 2 Division 1 occlusion come between these two extremes, with some discrepancy between upper and lower lips in the vertical dimension, though not enough to have an adverse effect on treatment.

The tongue function in Class 2 Division 1 occlusion occasionally imposes limitations on treatment. As has been described in Chapter 5, adaptive postural and functional positions of the tongue do not

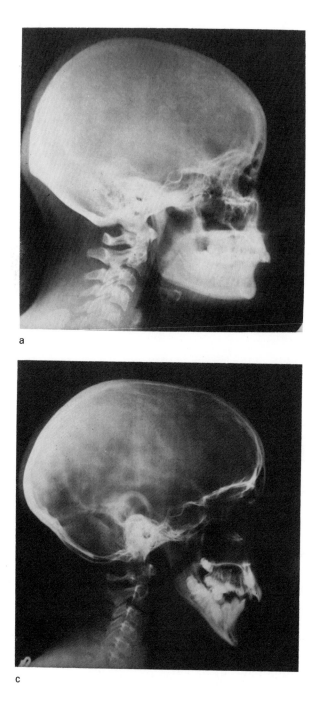

a

c

17.1. Variation in Class 2 Division 1 occlusion. Variation can be seen in the degree of Class 2 relationship, the inclination of the incisor teeth, the overjet and the overbite.

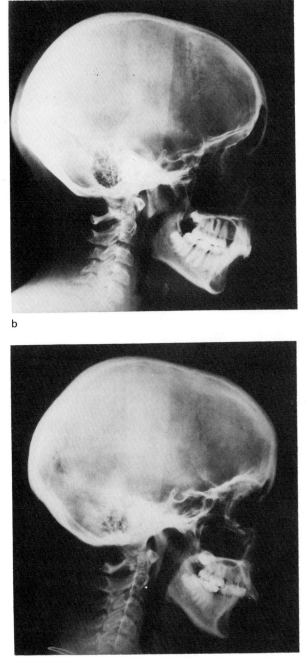

b

d

Fig. 17.1. (*cont*). Variation in Class 2 Division 1 occlusion.

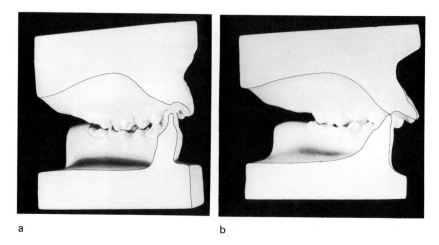

a   b

Fig. 17.2. Variation in incisal overbite in Class 2 Division 1 occlusion.

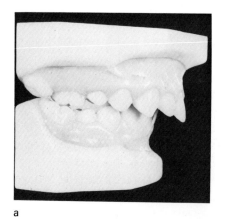

a

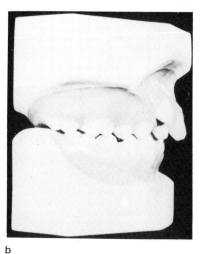

b

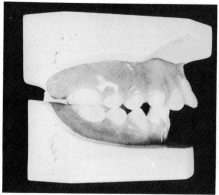

c

Fig. 17.3. Variation in crowding and in arch relationship in Class 2 Division 1 occlusion.

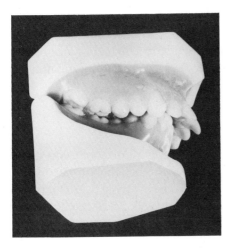

Fig. 17.4. Models of Class 2 Division 1 occlusion, the lower arch being too narrow for the upper.

normally cause problems in treatment, since alteration of tooth position takes away the need for adaptive tongue positions, but the endogenous forward positioning of the tongue may not be altered by changes in tooth position and may eventually reproduce open bites of Class 2 incisor relationships after treatment is completed. Fortunately, although it is not possible to distinguish with certainty between adaptive and endogenous function, problems caused by the latter are uncommon.

The size of the dentition in relation to jaw size is also variable, and may affect the treatment plan, though this factor does not normally limit corrective treatment. Ideally, there is enough space in the jaws for all the teeth to be accommodated in their correct positions and relationships, in which case the only problems are those caused by skeletal and muscle factors. Frequently, however, the dentition is too large for the jaws, a situation which may have been aggravated by extraction of primary teeth. The crowding problem is then superimposed on the problem of the Class 2 relationship.

Crowding of the upper teeth is often masked in Class 2 Division 1 occlusion by the increase in size of the dental arch brought about by the proclination of the incisors, and treatment to reduce the dental arch size usually necessitates a reduction in the dentition. Similarly, a lower dental arch which appears to be uncrowded in the adolescent may not have enough space for the third molars to be accommodated in early adult life.

By and large, the major aetiological factors which have been discussed produce most of the variation seen in Class 2 Division 1 occlusion. The wide range of possibilities produced by these factors cannot be described here, but will readily be envisaged. In addition, more localized factors such as have been discussed in Chapter 7 can play a part in altering the position of the teeth. The importance of assessing all the factors involved, and their severity, before formulating a treatment plan, cannot be over-emphasized.

Treatment objectives in Class 2 Division 1

The objectives of treatment in Class 2 Division 1 occlusion depend on the prevailing occlusal condition and the aetiological factors. In most cases, a complete correction of the excessive incisal overjet is possible. In some, reduction of excessive overbite will be necessary. It may be desirable to correct the Class 2 relationship of the buccal teeth, though this is not always considered to be necessary. In some cases, however, at the extremes of the range of normal variation, skeletal and muscular factors are such that full correction is not possible, and treatment objectives need to be modified. In such cases, excessive overjet and overbite may have to be accepted or corrected by surgical procedures. It is usually possible to correct crowding by the removal of teeth, and local irregularities can also usually be corrected by orthodontic treatment.

The objectives of treatment may therefore include:
1 Relief of crowding and local irregularities.
2 Reduction of incisal overbite.
3 Reduction of incisal overjet.
4 Correction of Class 2 relationship of the buccal teeth.

Crowding and local irregularities are not specific to Class 2 occlusions, and have been considered in previous chapters. Only those treatment principles relevant to Class 2 Division 1 occlusion will be considered here.

Treatment in Class 2 Division 1

Although the most obvious result of Class 2 treatment is the change in upper incisor position, it is probably true to say that the key to successful treatment lies in the correct position of the lower incisal arch and the canine relationship. Given a stable and uncrowded lower incisal arch, if it is possible to produce a correct relationship between upper and lower canines it should be possible to produce a correct incisor relationship and a satisfactory relationship of the buccal teeth. The lower arch holds the key to successful treatment by virtue of the fact that the major factors which govern final tooth stability, i.e. the lower lip, the tongue and mandibular function, are all directly associated with the position of the lower teeth.

The lower dental arch

A stable lower incisor position must be judged taking into account the axial inclination of the incisors and the muscular relationship of the incisal arch, i.e. the position of the tongue and lower lip. Many patients with Class 2 Division 1 occlusion do not need any change in the general position of the lower incisal arch except for the reduction of the vertical dimension in excessive overbite and the correction of irregularities due to crowding. Others, whose lower incisors have been retroclined by thumb sucking or by lip activity may need some proclination of these teeth as part of corrective treatment. It is unusual for retroclination of lower incisors to be required in Class 2 treatment.

Thus one of the first steps in treatment planning in Class 2 Division 1 is consideration of the lower dental arch. The arch may be:
1 Completely satisfactory in position and form.
2 Crowded, in which case teeth will need to be removed.
3 Spaced, in which case the buccal teeth may be moved forward during treatment.
4 The incisors may be retroclined, and it may be possible to procline them as part of treatment to reduce the overjet.
5 There may be excessive vertical development of the incisal arch, giving excessive overbite which needs reduction during treatment.

There may, of course, be any combination of these features. Some examples of these lower arch features are shown in Figs. 17.2–17.4.

The upper dental arch

By definition, the incisal overjet is excessive and this is usually, though not invariably, associated with proclination of the upper incisors. The upper arch may be spaced, crowded or regular. The relationship of the buccal teeth to the lower arch is variable, ranging from a mild Class 2 relationship of the buccal teeth, in which case the upper incisors are likely to be spaced or the lower incisors crowded, to a severe degree of Class 2 relationship.

The treatment required will reflect the conditions of the dental arches as well as the degree of skeletal discrepancy. Treatment principles will be considered under the headings of extractions, reduction of overbite, reduction of overjet and correction of buccal segment relationships.

Extractions in Class 2 Division 1 treatment

Extraction of teeth has three main functions:

1   To relieve crowding in either arch.

2   To provide space in the upper arch for the retraction of the anterior segment.

3   To provide space in the lower arch for intermaxillary traction.

In a mild Class 2 relationship with a satisfactory lower arch form, no lower extractions may be necessary, since the upper arch can usually be treated by intra-maxillary and extra-oral traction. It may even be possible to carry out treatment without upper extractions if the buccal teeth are in Class 1 relationship and the upper incisors are spaced (Fig. 17.5). This situation is unusual in British populations, though more common in Central and Eastern European populations, where inter-maxillary traction with functional appliances is frequently the treatment of choice.

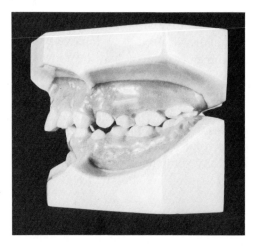

Fig. 17.5. Class 1 occlusion of the buccal teeth, with excessive overjet and spacing of upper incisors caused by lip and tongue activity. As the buccal teeth are in correct relationship, reduction of the overjet should be possible without extractions.

The teeth most frequently extracted in Class 2 treatment are the first premolars, since they provide space in the most convenient position, i.e. in the centre of each quadrant of the dental arches. Generally speaking, the removal of any other teeth provides complications to treatment, although, in a very crowded jaw, it is sometimes necessary to remove two teeth on each side of the upper arch to give space to relieve crowding and to reduce the incisal overjet.

Reduction of overbite

If the incisal overbite is excessive it is not possible to reduce the overjet completely without first reducing the overbite. Reduction of overbite is therefore a frequent part of Class 2 Division 1 treatment, and is usually carried out as one of the first stages.

There are three ways of reducing overbite:

1   by using an anterior bite plane on an upper removable appliance (see Chapter 13);
2   by using a lower fixed appliance to apply direct downward force to the lower incisors;
3   by using an upper fixed appliance to apply direct upward force to the upper incisors.

As far as is known, the anterior bite plane causes reduction in overbite by allowing vertical development of the posterior dento-alveolar segments (Menezes 1975). There is some evidence that fixed appliances may reduce overbite by causing intrusion of the anterior segments, at least in the short-term, as well as by allowing vertical development of the posterior segments. It seems likely that, in the long-term, permanent reduction of overbite is associated with vertical growth of the jaws.

Reduction of overjet

Overjet reduction is usually brought about by retraction of the anterior segment of the upper arch. Since this reduces the size of the arch, it can only be carried out if there is adequate space for tooth movement. Occasionally, overjet reduction may be achieved by moving the lower incisors forward or by moving the whole upper arch backward, though, it is unusual to find conditions in which these movements produce stable results.

The method used for retraction of the upper incisors depends essentially on the degree of Class 2 skeletal discrepancy. If the discrepancy is mild, a simple tipping movement of the incisors should be sufficient to produce a satisfactory incisor relationship. This can be brought about by a removable appliance using intra-maxillary traction if the increase in overjet is not severe (see Figs. 13.3 and 13.9). Anchorage may be reinforced with extra-oral traction, or fixed appliances using inter-maxillary traction may be used if the overjet is large and a considerable tipping movement is necessary (Fig. 14.9).

The more severe the skeletal Class 2 discrepancy, the less satisfactory simple tipping movements become in reducing overjet. This is because a severe Class 2 skeletal pattern would necessitate excessive retroclination of the upper incisors to bring about full correction of the overjet (see Fig. 9.10). Therefore, in the more severe skeletal discrepancies, it is necessary to produce bodily movement of the incisors to reduce the

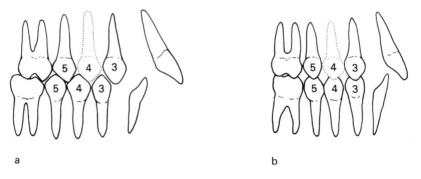

Fig. 17.6. (a) In Class 2 Division 1 occlusion, when extraction in the upper arch leaves only just enough space to retract the upper canine into a Class 1 relationship, reinforced anchorage, such as extra oral anchorage, is necessary to avoid space loss. (b) When the upper arch extraction leaves more than enough space to achieve a Class 1 canine relationship, reinforced anchorage is not so important.

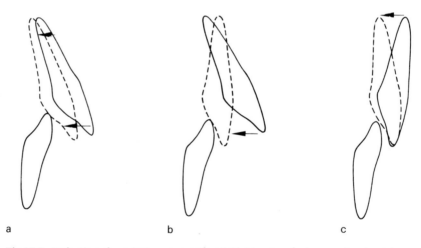

Fig 17.7. Reduction of overjet in a severe Class 2 Division 1 occlusion may involve (a) bodily movement of incisors; or (b) tipping; followed by (c) apical torquing movement.

overjet without producing excessive retroclination. This can either be done by direct bodily movement or by tipping followed by apical torque (Fig. 17.7).

Ideally, overjet reduction will bring about a normal incisor relationship. However, the essential feature of stability following treatment is that the incisors must be in balance between the muscular forces acting on them. This means that the overjet must be reduced to such an extent that the lower lip functions in front of the upper incisors. This may sometimes occur without there being an ideal incisor relationship. (See also page 104.)

Correction of buccal segment relationships

Whether it is necessary to produce Class 1 relationship of the buccal teeth in the treatment of Class 2 Division 1 occlusion is a debatable point. More generally accepted is the desirability of producing good functional occlusion of the buccal teeth. Whether this is best achieved by producing cuspal interdigitation is also debatable, but in the absence of good evidence to the contrary cuspal interdigitation is usually preferred to cusp-to-cusp contacts. Thus the objective of treatment in the buccal segments is to correct cusp-to-cusp contacts such as are shown in Fig. 17.3c. This can be done either by producing Class 1 relationships or Class 2 relationships of a whole premolar unit in degree (Fig. 17.8). There are three basic ways of achieving this.

1 Distal movement of upper buccal teeth. This will produce Class 1 relationship, but can only be done if the jaw is large enough to accommodate the teeth in a more distal position. It can be achieved with the use of extra-oral traction, sometimes after the extraction of the upper second molars (Fig. 17.8a), or with intermaxillary traction using functional appliances (Fig. 17.8b).

2 Mesial movement of lower buccal teeth. This will also produce Class 1 relationship. It is frequently carried out following removal of a premolar from each side of the upper and lower jaws. Intermaxillary traction is applied to move the upper anterior segment back and the lower posterior segment forward (Fig. 17.8b). Spontaneous movement after extraction of first premolars is seldom enough to correct Class 2 molar relationships. (Stephens & Lloyd 1980).

3 Mesial movement of upper buccal teeth. This produces Class 2 relationship with cuspal interdigitation, and is appropriate to the less severe Class 2 Division 1 occlusion where the lower arch is satisfactory. An upper premolar is extracted on each side of the jaw. The upper anterior segment is moved back and the upper posterior segment forward into the extraction space using intra-maxillary traction (Fig. 17.8c).

It is not appropriate to discuss here all the variations on these basic treatments of the buccal segment relationship. The treatment of choice mainly depends on the degree of Class 2 discrepancy and the degree of crowding, which must include the presence of third molars. If third molars are present the lower arch frequently requires the extraction of teeth in the treatment of Class 2 Division 1 occlusion.

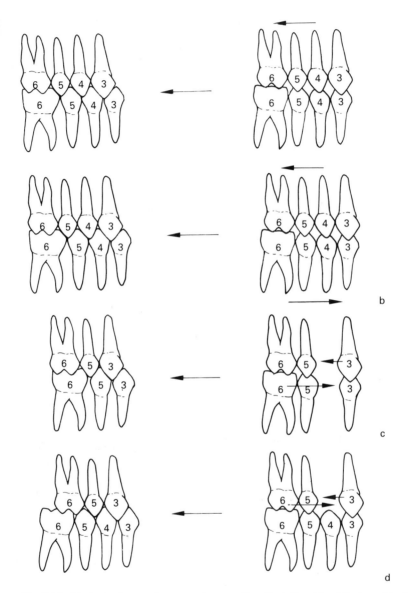

Fig. 17.8. Methods of correcting a cusp-to-cusp Class 2 relationship of the buccal teeth. (a) Distal movement of upper buccal teeth. (b) Intermaxillary traction without extractions. (c) Removal of upper and lower first premolars, intermaxillary traction to close extraction spaces. (d) Removal of upper premolars only, if no lower crowding present. Intramaxillary traction closes the extraction space and corrects the Class 2 relationship of the anterior teeth.

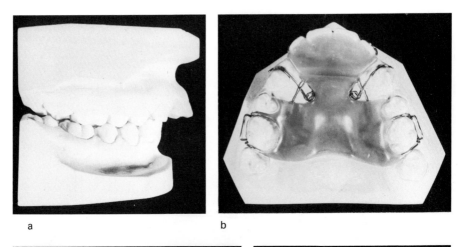

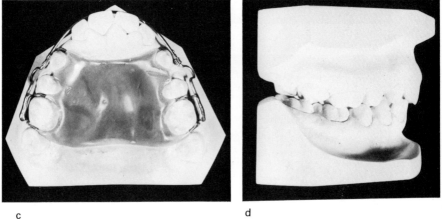

Fig. 17.9. Stages in treatment of a mild Class 2 Division 1 occlusion, using removable upper appliances. (a) Original occlusion. (b) Appliance to retract upper canine teeth after removal of upper first premolars. (c) Appliance to retrocline upper incisors. (d) Final occlusion.

Figs. 17.9 and 17.10 show stages in the treatment of a mild and a more severe Class 2 Division 1 occlusion, illustrating some of the principles previously discussed.

TIMING OF TREATMENT

The timing of treatment in Class 2 Division 1 occlusion depends on the type of treatment required. When no extractions are necessary, treatment with functional appliances is often carried out in the mixed dentition, before premolars and permanent canines erupt. If extractions are

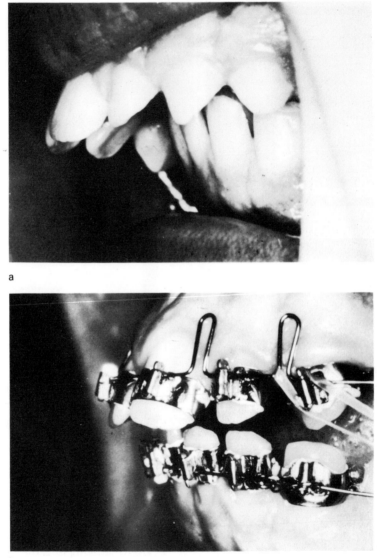

Fig. 17.10. Stages in treatment of a severe Class 2 Division 1 occlusion using multiband fixed appliances. (a) Original occlusion. (b) Intermaxillary traction following removal of first premolars. (c) Apical torque to move back upper incisor roots. (d) Final occlusion.

needed, it is usual to carry out all the treatment after premolars and permanent canines erupt.

In some children, with severe proclination of the upper incisors, early reduction of the incisal overjet has been advocated, since proclined

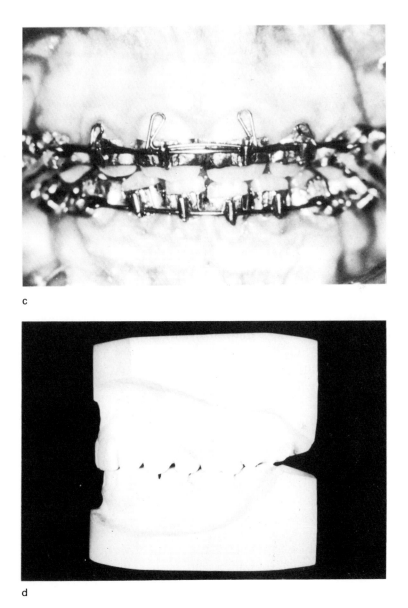

c

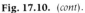

d

Fig. 17.10. (*cont*).

incisors are thought to be vulnerable to accidental trauma. However, it is often not possible to achieve full reduction of the overjet without making space by extraction of teeth, and therefore a two-stage treatment would be required, i.e. partial reduction of the overjet in the mixed dentition, followed later by extraction of premolar teeth and completion of treatment. Retention appliances would need to be worn between the two stages. Even partial reduction of the overjet is only possible if space is available in the upper anterior segment, otherwise the unerupted permanent upper canine teeth would interfere with tooth movement. For these reasons, early reduction of the incisal overjet, though desirable, is often not practicable except with the use of functional appliances.

The timing of orthodontic treatment in relation to puberal growth will be discussed in Chapter 19. It has been suggested that orthodontic tooth movement may progress more rapidly during the puberal growth spurt, and that treatment should be timed accordingly. At present there is little evidence on this matter, but several investigations are in progress.

Class 2 Division 2 occlusion

Much that has been said about the Class 2 Division 1 applies equally to the Class 2 Division 2 occlusion. The basic causes of variation are the same. The role of extractions in treatment, and the correction of the buccal segment relationship are essentially the same. There are, however, certain differences with regard to incisor positions and their correction which will be outlined here.

The features of Class 2 Division 2 occlusion

The Class 2 relationship of the dental arches, combined with retroclination of the upper incisors and excessive incisal overbite, are the essential features of this type of occlusion. The skeletal relationship and dental arch crowding are just as variable as in Class 2 Division 1 occlusion, but the muscle factors show less variation.

There is usually a low gonial angle, giving a rather square facial profile. In most cases, the lips have sufficient vertical dimension to be able to meet in the rest position, and, in spite of any horizontal skeletal Class 2 discrepancy, the lips meet in front of the upper central incisors. The greater the skeletal discrepancy, therefore, the more retroclined the upper central incisors are likely to be. The level at which the upper and lower lips meet is usually high on the labial surface of the upper incisors. If there is crowding of the upper dental arch, the upper lateral incisors or canines may be proclined in front of the lower lip function. There is commonly a pronounced labio-mental groove beneath the lower lip.

Fig. 17.11. illustrates these facial and dental characteristics of Class 2 Division 2 occlusion.

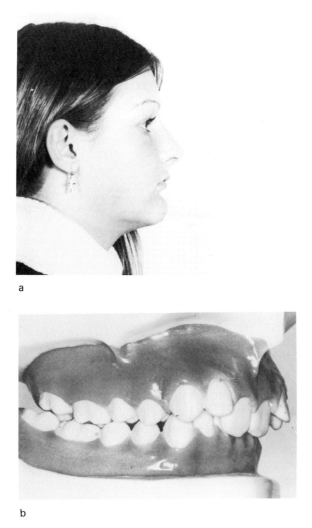

a

b

Fig. 17.11. Facial and dental characteristics of Class 2 Division 2 occlusion.

THE INCISOR POSITIONS IN CLASS 2 DIVISION 2

The retroclination of the incisors and the deep incisal overbite are among the main features which warrant treatment in Class 2 Division 2 occlusion. The deep overbite may result in gingival trauma both on the palatal gingivae in the upper jaw and the labial gingivae in the lower jaw. Although it has been suggested that the deep overbite may be a result of excessive vertical development of the anterior dento-alveolar segments, Mills (1973) has shown that excessive development does not occur in the milder antero-posterior skeletal discrepancies, and that deep overbite is simply a result of retroclination of the incisors. It was also associated with relatively small lower facial height. In the more severe skeletal Class 2 discrepancies, however, where there is no contact between upper and lower incisor teeth, it is possible that excessive vertical development of the anterior segments occurs, and in such cases the overbite may be very deep (Fig. 7.25).

The incisal overjet is not usually increased except in the more severe Class 2 skeletal relationships.

Treatment objectives and limitations

The possible objectives of treatment in Class 2 Division 2 occlusion can be listed as follows.

1   Relief of crowding and local irregularities.
2   Relief of anterior gingival trauma, and correction of incisal inclinations.
3   Correction of buccal segment relationships.

The relief of crowding and local irregularities has been discussed previously.

Correction of buccal segment relationships is much the same as outlined for Class 2 Division 1 occlusion, except that inter- and intramaxillary traction is not aimed at reducing incisal overjet.

The relief of anterior gingival trauma necessitates movement of the incisor teeth to a position where the lower incisor contacts the palatal surface of the upper incisor in occlusion. This can only be brought about by reduction of the inter-incisal angle.

The limiting factors to this treatment are the musculature of the lower lip and the degree of Class 2 skeletal discrepancy. If the lower lip line is high, proclination of the upper anterior segment by simple tipping movements is not possible. If there is a severe Class 2 skeletal relationship the lower anterior segment cannot be proclined sufficiently to meet the upper teeth (Fig. 17.12).

Principles of treatment of incisor relationships

In a mild Class 2 Division 2 relationship, where there is no gingival trauma, it is usual to accept the relationship of the central incisors and simply to relieve any crowding by extraction of teeth and to correct local irregularities.

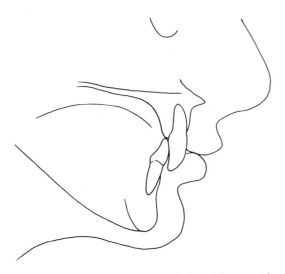

Fig. 17.12. In Class 2 Division 2 occlusion with severe Class 2 skeletal relationship the lower incisors cannot be proclined sufficiently to achieve normal contact with the upper incisors.

When gingival trauma exists, more extensive corrective treatment with multiband fixed appliances is needed. As far as the incisor relationships are concerned, this treatment consists of:

1 Reduction of incisal overbite.
2 Alteration of incisal inclinations to achieve stable incisal contacts.

Reduction of incisal overbite can be brought about by using an upper anterior bite plane or an upper or lower fixed appliance, as for Class 2 Division 1 treatment. Mills (1973) has suggested that overbite reduction in Class 2 Division 2 treatment does not occur by intrusion of the anterior teeth but is associated with vertical growth of the lower face.

Alteration of incisal inclinations usually involves the use of torquing movement to move the incisal apices in a lingual direction. Proclination by tipping the incisor crowns forward tends to relapse because of pressure from the lower lip, particularly in the upper arch. Some proclination of the lower incisors, after reducing the overbite, may be stable (Fig. 17.13).

In the younger patient in the late mixed dentition, with active growth still to be completed, it may be possible to procline the upper incisors, effectively converting the occlusion to Class 2 Division 1, and then to use a functional appliance to correct the Class 2 relationship. This procedure is likely to be more successful in the absence of marked crowding of the dentition.

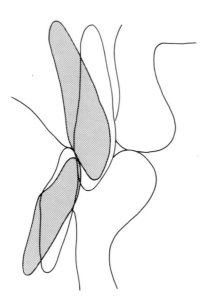

Fig. 17.13. Class 2 Division 2 occlusion. Alteration of the incisal inclinations to achieve a normal overbite involves root torque and vertical movements.

THE SEVERE CLASS 2 DIVISION 2

When the Class 2 Division 2 occlusion is based on a severe Class 2 skeletal discrepancy, full corrective orthodontic treatment may be impossible. In such cases, gingival trauma may be relieved by first reducing the incisal overbite and then maintaining the new tooth positions with a permanent retention appliance. Provided the buccal teeth are in occlusion, an upper anterior bite plane on a removable cast metal base is a satisfactory method of maintaining incisor positions. With any such permanent appliance, of course, the general health of the oral tissues must receive special attention.

Summary

Class 2 occlusions include all the localized occlusal problems, and have the added problem of Class 2 dental arch relationship.

Class 2 Division 1 occlusion

1   The main variants within this classification are:
   - The degree of Class 2 discrepancy.
   - The inclination of the incisors and the degree of overjet.

- The degree of incisal overbite.
- The degree of crowding.

2   These variations are brought about by variation in:
- The skeletal relationship.
- Muscle form and function.
- The size of the dentition and the size of the jaws.

3   Treatment objectives include:
- Relief of crowding and local irregularities.
- Reduction of incisal overbite.
- Reduction of incisal overjet.
- Correction of buccal segment relationships.

TREATMENT

Treatment should be planned around a stable position of the lower incisal arch, since the functional mechanisms controlling tooth position are closely related to the lower anterior segment.

Extraction of teeth is often necessary and has the following purposes:

1   To relieve crowding.

2   To provide space in the upper arch for retraction of the anterior segment, possibly for protraction of the posterior segment.

3   To provide space in the lower arch for inter-maxillary traction.

The first premolars are most frequently removed for these purposes.

Reduction of overbite, if necessary, is brought about by the use of an upper anterior bite plane or by fixed appliances which may achieve some intrusion of the incisors.

Reduction of overjet may be achieved by:

1   Retraction of the upper arch with extra-oral forces.

2   Retraction of the upper arch and protraction of the lower arch with inter-maxillary forces, e.g. functional appliances.

3   Retraction of the upper anterior segment into natural or extraction spaces, with intra-maxillary or intermaxillary traction forces.

4   Protraction of the lower anterior segment.

For these movements to be successful there must be adequate space in the jaws and the final positions of the teeth must be in muscle balance. A Class 1 relationship of the upper and lower canines is a prerequisite for correct incisor relationships.

Correction of buccal segment relationships may be achieved by:

1   Distal movement of upper buccal teeth, producing a Class 1 relationship.

2 Mesial movement of lower buccal teeth, possibly into extraction spaces, producing Class 1 relationship.
3 Mesial movement of upper buccal teeth into extraction spaces, producing Class 2 relationship with cuspal interdigitation.

Class 2 Division 2 occlusion

The main features include a low gonial angle, high lip line, retroclined incisors and excessive incisal overbite.

The main differences between Class 2 Division 1 and Division 2 treatment lie in the correction of the incisor positions.

Treatment objectives include:
1 Relief of crowding and local irregularities.
2 Relief of anterior gingival trauma and correction of incisal inclinations.
3 Correction of buccal segment relationships.

Limitations to correction of incisor relationships are the musculature of the lower lip and the degree of Class 2 skeletal discrepancy.

TREATMENT OF INCISOR RELATIONSHIPS

In a mild Class 2 Division 2, with no gingival trauma, treatment may be confined to correction of crowding and local irregularities.

When gingival trauma exists, treatment includes:
1 Reduction of incisal overbite with anterior bite plane or fixed appliances.
2 Alteration of incisal inclinations to achieve contact between upper and lower incisors, usually with fixed appliances.

Proclination of upper incisors is not usually successful owing to lip pressure, and apical torque may be necessary.

In the younger patient, proclination of upper incisor followed by functional appliance treatment may be successful.

A severe Class 2 skeletal discrepancy may prevent the attainment of incisal contact, and, if there is gingival trauma, a permanent retainer may be necessary after reduction of overbite.

References

Foster, T. D. & Day, A. J. W. (1974) A survey of malocclusion and the need for orthodontic treatment in a Shropshire school population. *B J Orthod*, **1**, 73–78.

Menezes, D. M. (1975) Changes in the dento-facial complex as a result of bite plane therapy. *Am J Orthod*, **67**, 660–676.

Mills, J. R. E. (1973) The problem of overbite in Class II Division 2 occlusion. *Br J Orthod*, **1**, 34–38.

Stephens, C. D. & Lloyd, T. G. (1980) Changes in molar occlusion after extraction of all first premolars: a follow-up study of Class II Division I cases treated with removable appliances. *Br J Orthod*, **7**, 139–144.

Principles of treatment in Class 3 occlusal relationship

Class 3 is the least common type of occlusal relationship in many communities, occurring in less than 5% of individuals in British populations (Haynes 1970; Foster & Day 1974). It is therefore seen relatively infrequently in orthodontic practice, but can present some of the most difficult treatment problems. Indeed, it is probably true to say that a greater proportion of Class 3 occlusions are beyond correction by orthodontic treatment than is the case with Class 2 occlusions.

Apart from localized features, the main variants in Class 3 occlusions are as follows (Fig. 18.1):

1 The degree of Class 3 antero-posterior relationship of the dental arches.
2 The degree of lateral discrepancy in upper and lower dental arch size.
3 The degree of incisal overbite or anterior open bite.
4 The degree of crowding of the teeth.

As in all occlusions, the source of these variations is found in the main aetiological features, i.e. skeletal factors, the oral musculature and the size of the dentition. The influence of these features in Class 3 occlusions can be described as follows.

Skeletal factors

These play a major part in most Class 3 occlusions. Three important aspects of the skeletal form affect the occlusal relationships (Fig. 18.2).

1   The antero-posterior skeletal relationship

Almost all Class 3 occlusions are based on some degree of Class 3 skeletal relationship. The antero-posterior skeletal discrepancy is largely responsible for the Class 3 occlusal relationship and the reversed overjet and in many cases the buccal crossbite.

2   The relative widths of upper and lower jaws

Unilateral or bilateral crossbite may be caused by discrepancy in width of the jaws. Similarly, since the buccal segments diverge towards the back,

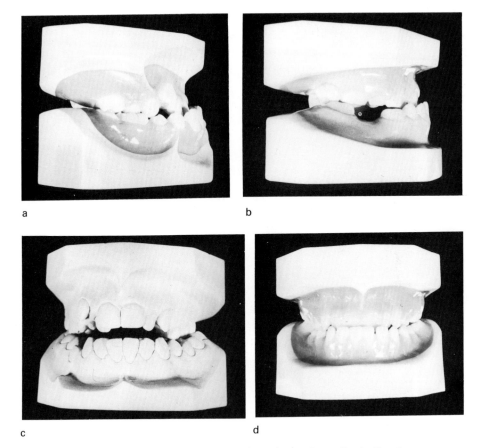

Fig. 18.1. Variation in overbite, overjet, buccal crossbite and crowding in Class 3 occlusion.

discrepancy in antero-posterior relationship may produce crossbite. (See Chapter 7).

3   The vertical dimension of the face

The height of the lower part of the face is made up by the height of the teeth and of the jaws. It is also influenced by the gonial angle of the mandible, a high gonial angle tending to give a long face, and a low gonial angle tending to give a short face in the vertical dimension. This may be reflected in the occlusal relationship by variation in the incisal overbite, the short face tending to have a deep overbite and the long face an anterior open bite.

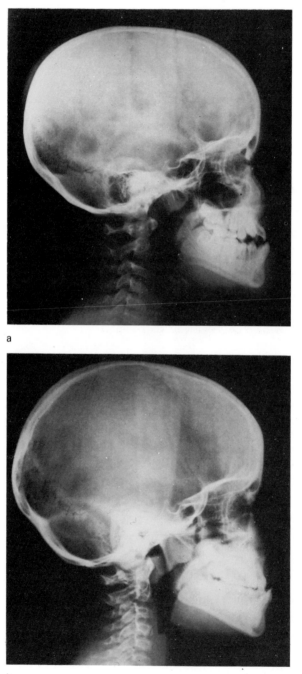

a

b

Fig. 18.2. Variation in skeletal form in Class 3 occlusion.

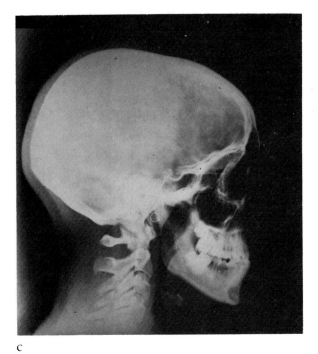

c

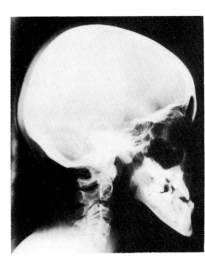

d

Fig. 18.2. *(cont).*

All these skeletal features are continuous variants, and, to a large extent, determine the severity of the occlusal problem. They also provide the main limiting factors to corrective treatment.

The oral musculature

In contrast to the Class 2 occlusion, variation in lip form and function plays little part in variation in Class 3 occlusions. While the vertical and antero-posterior relationships of the upper and lower lips vary with lip size and with skeletal relationship, these variations do not seem to be reflected to any great extent in variations in tooth position. There is a tendency for the lower incisors to be more retroclined than in other occlusal relationships, possible due to lower lip function in conjunction with the skeletal discrepancy.

The tongue, being attached to the inner border of the lower jaw, usually matches the lower dental arch in size. If the upper arch is much smaller than the lower arch, the tongue, by virtue of its size and function, may play a part in producing an anterior open bite. It may also limit corrective treatment, as will be seen later.

The size of the dentition

This is a continuous variant, as in all occlusions. In the Class 3 relationship it is unusual to find crowding of the lower teeth since the lower jaw is not normally small. In the larger lower jaws the lower teeth may be spaced. Crowding of the upper jaw, on the other hand, is common, though not invariable.

Thus, it can be seen that the skeletal, muscular and dental factors can produce Class 3 occlusions with a wide range of variation. It is usually necessary, in assessment, to differentiate between discrepancies in the *size* and in the *position* of the upper and lower jaws. Discrepancy in size is often present, with the lower jaw being larger than the upper. This will be manifested as a difference in the crowding or spacing condition between the two dental arches. Discrepancy in position between the jaws is also often present, particularly in the sagittal and vertical planes, the sagittal discrepancy often producing crossbite in the transverse dimension. Two extreme types of Class 3 occlusion have been described, one having a small maxilla and a high gonial angle and the other having a maxilla of more normal size, a large mandible and a low gonial angle. This concept has received some support. Jones (1975) found a significant relationship between the length of the maxilla and the gonial angle in Class 3 occlusions, the short maxilla being related to the high gonial angle. There are, however, many intermediate types which do not fit neatly into any classification. One type which seems to stand out from the others is the postural or displacement Class 3, which has been mentioned in Chapter 2 (see Fig. 2.11). In this type of occlusion, which is based on a mild Class 3 skeletal relationship, the incisor positions are such that the upper and lower incisal edges meet in initial contact when the mandible is closing. There is a translocated forward closure of the mandible from the rest to the occlusal position, the lower incisors being in front of the upper incisors in occlusion. The upper incisors are usually retroclined. Postural Class 3 occlusion is uncommon, probably occurring in less than 0.5% of individuals in British populations (Foster & Day 1974).

Treatment objectives and limitations

The main treatment objectives in Class 3 occlusion may include:
1   Reduction of crowding.
2   Correction of the reversed overjet.
3   Correction of incisal overbite.
4   Correction of buccal segment relationship.

Reduction of crowding is more often necessary in the upper jaw than in the lower, and follows the principles of extraction of teeth previously outlined. If the reversed overjet is to be corrected, it is usually better to delay extractions in the upper arch until a stable incisor position has been achieved.

Correction of reversed overjet

The major limiting factors to the correction of reversed overjet are the antero-posterior skeletal relationship of the jaws, the presence of anterior open bite and the tongue. Reversed overjet could be corrected by moving the upper incisors forward or the lower incisors back. In the more severe skeletal Class 3 discrepancies, the incisor teeth cannot be moved sufficiently to overcome the effects of the dental base relationship. Even if the teeth can be moved sufficiently to produce correct antero-posterior relationships, they will not be maintained in that position without a positive incisal overbite (Fig. 18.3). Finally, the tongue may prevent any retroclination of the lower incisors during treatment, and thus limit corrective treatment.

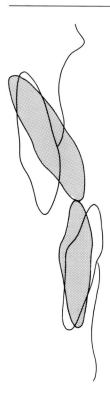

Fig. 18.3. In Class 3 occlusion with a severe skeletal discrepancy, tilting of the incisors is unlikely to produce a positive overbite.

Correction of incisal overbite

The incisal overbite may be excessively deep, or, at the other extreme, there may be anterior open bite. Correction of deep overbite depends entirely on correction of reversed overjet. If the incisors can be placed in correct antero-posterior relationship during the growth period, vertical development of the buccal dento-alveolar segments should bring about a normal overbite relationship. At the end of the growth period this is less likely to happen, and the patient may be left with incisal contact only, the buccal teeth remaining out of occlusion.

Correction of anterior open bite is much more difficult, and is limited by the size and function of the tongue and the vertical dimension of the face. A minor degree of anterior open bite may be corrected by producing vertical movement of upper and lower incisor teeth, but with any major discrepancy, orthodontic treatment may not be sufficient to overcome the limiting factors.

Correction of buccal segment relationships

Antero-posterior buccal segment relationships can be corrected, if thought necessary, by movement of segments or of individual teeth into extraction spaces, similar to that described for Class 2 relationship. The difference in Class 3 relationship is that upper buccal teeth would need to be moved forward and lower buccal teeth backward. Again, the limiting factor is the degree of antero-posterior skeletal discrepancy, and it is often thought unnecessary to correct buccal segment relationships.

The correction of lateral buccal segment relationships, unilateral or bilateral crossbites, is not always considered necessary. Generally speaking, it is thought desirable to correct unilateral crossbites which involve initial contact and translocated closure of the mandible, and this correction is readily achieved by expansion of the upper dental arch. Bilateral crossbites, which are symmetrical, and in which mandibular closure is not deviated, are often accepted. The limiting factor to their correction is the relative narrowness of the upper dental base, though techniques of rapid maxillary expansion are sometimes used to overcome this when it is thought necessary (see Chapter 7).

Principles of treatment

From the previous sections it can be seen that the factors which are of most importance in planning treatment in Class 3 occlusion are:
1 The skeletal relationship, incisal inclinations and overjet.
2 The incisal overbite.
3 The form and function of the tongue.
4 The crowding and spacing condition of the dental arches.
Assessment of the skeletal relationship, incisal inclinations and overjet will show whether it is possible to achieve a correct incisor relationship by simple tipping of the teeth, upper or lower, or both, whether bodily movement or apical torque is necessary, or whether the problem is beyond the scope of orthodontic treatment.

Assessment of the incisal overbite will show whether any vertical movement of the teeth is necessary to achieve a positive overbite, which is essential for the stability of a correct incisor relationship. It must be remembered that simple tipping movements tend to reduce the incisal overbite. If a severe anterior open bite is present, the problem may again be beyond correction by orthodontic treatment alone.

Assessment of tongue form and function will show whether the lower incisors can be retroclined in treatment and whether there is any physical barrier to correction of an anterior open bite.

Finally, crowding or spacing must be assessed. Crowding will normally be reduced by extraction of teeth, but in Class 3 occlusions crowding in the upper arch may be relieved, at least in part, by the increase in arch size which occurs when the upper anterior segment is moved forward during treatment. It is usual, therefore, to delay extractions, if possible until the anterior segment is in its final stable position. Crowding in the lower arch is unusual, but theoretically, lower teeth need to be extracted if the lower arch is to be made smaller during treatment. This does not apply if spacing exists in the lower arch, as it often does in a Class 3 occlusion with a large mandible.

Treatment in mild and postural Class 3 relationships

When the skeletal discrepancy is slight, and there is a positive incisal overbite, proclination of the upper anterior teeth and relief of crowding is often the only orthodontic treatment necessary. This is usually the case in postural Class 3 occlusions, in which the upper incisors are retroclined. The forward movement of the upper incisors removes the initial contact during mandibular closure, and allows the mandible to resume its correct occlusal relationship with the maxilla. It is necessary to 'unlock' the incisor occlusion to allow the upper incisors to be moved across the line of the lower arch. This is done by adding posterior bite planes to the appliance.

Appliances for proclination of the upper anterior teeth are shown in Figs. 13.4 and 13.10.

In some circumstances, depending on the axial inclination of the incisor teeth, retroclination of the lower incisors may be a more appropriate form of treatment than proclination of the upper incisors. There must be sufficient space in the arch for this movement, and the limitations imposed by the tongue must be borne in mind.

Treatment in moderate Class 3 relationship

When the skeletal discrepancy is more severe, tipping of one anterior segment is unlikely to produce enough movement to correct the incisor relationship. It will probably be necessary to move the upper teeth forward and the lower teeth back. This can be brought about by intermaxillary traction, in this case usually known as reversed intermaxillary traction or Class 3 traction. Although it can be carried out with removable appliances, it is better managed with fixed appliances, which will also serve to correct the incisal overbite if necessary (Fig. 18.4). Extra-oral traction forces can also be applied to the lower arch (Orton *et al.* 1983).

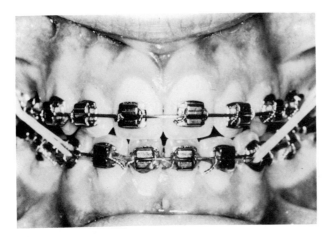

Fig. 18.4. Inter-maxillary traction to correct Class 3 occlusion.

It may be necessary to achieve bodily movement of the anterior teeth to overcome the skeletal discrepancy, either directly or by means of tipping followed by apical torque.

Early treatment with functional appliances may often be successful (Loh & Kerr 1985).

RETENTION AFTER TREATMENT

Although a period of mechanical retention of tooth position after active treatment is necessary after rotations, vertical movements and other local tooth movment, it is not usually necessary to retain the incisor positions after correction of reversed overjet. Provided an adequate incisal overbite has been achieved, the occlusion of upper and lower incisors is normally sufficient to maintain the new tooth positions with the forces of mastication. It is important that the buccal teeth are in occlusion before appliances are finally removed, otherwise the anterior teeth receive the full load of the masticatory forces and there may be subsequent damage to the periodontal supporting structures. It is very easy to produce traumatic incisor relationships in the more severe Class 3 occlusions, and the end result of such treatment may be worse than the original condition.

Severe Class 3 occlusion

A small number of Class 3 occlusions are beyond the limits of correction by orthodontic treatment alone. These are usually at the extremes of the normal range of mandibular prognathism, maxillary retrognathism or facial height. If it is felt necessary to apply corrective treatment in these cases, surgical repositioning of the jaws can be carried out. The discrepancy is likely to be three-dimensional, i.e. in the antero-posterior, transverse and vertical planes, and the soft tissue elements attached to the jaws, notably the tongue and the masticatory muscles, are also involved. Complex re-arrangement of the bony elements is therefore necessary if treatment is to be successful, and the basis of the re-arrangement is the dental occlusion. Orthodontic treatment is frequently a necessary part of the overall corrective treatment in these cases.

If it is not considered necessary or desirable to correct the Class 3 relationship, orthodontic treatment would be confined to the relief of any crowding and the alignment of any local irregularities in the dental arches.

Influence of growth on Class 3 treatment

It is generally considered that growth changes in Class 3 occlusal relationships are more likely to make the condition worse than better. Though there is individual variation, clinical experience suggests that, during growth, the mandible tends to become more prognathic than the maxilla, and in some Class 3 occlusions this growth change is very marked (Fig. 18.5). This view has received some support from the work of Silviera (1985) among others, while Lewis and Roche (1988) have reported that mandibular growth relative to the cranial base progresses after 17 years of age.

It is perhaps because of these progressive growth changes that there is a tendency for Class 3 treatments to be started in the mixed dentition. Many operators feel that, if the incisor relationship can be corrected at an early stage, further mandibular growth will cause the upper incisors to be moved forward through occlusal contact. There is no positive evidence to support this rationale of treatment, but it may be effective over minor growth changes. A major disparity between upper and lower jaw growth, however, is likely to overcome any early treatment, and it is not unusual to find that a normal overjet achieved during the mixed dentition phase is lost as the mandible grows more than the maxilla during adolescence.

Another reason put forward for early treatment is the suggestion that the form of the growing mandible may be altered, either by the forces of normal occlusion or by external forces applied at an early stage.

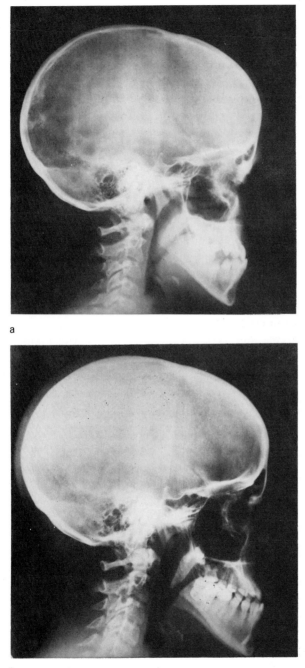

Fig. 18.5.   Class 3 skeletal relationship becoming more severe with growth. (a) 10 years.
(b) 13 years of age.

To this end, methods of treatment have been instituted aimed at modifying the shape of the mandible by applying external force through a chin-cap from occipital traction headgear (Sakamoto *et al.* 1984; Wendell 1984). The objective is to reduce the forward component of mandibular growth, and consequently the degree of Class 3 relationship. While such forces can certainly produce retroclination of the lower incisors, there is some doubt as to whether they can affect the growth of the basal part of the jaw, since they are not normally strong enough or constant enough to have a lasting effect.

Summary

The main variants in Class 3 occlusion are:
1   The antero-posterior dental arch relationship.
2   Lateral discrepancies in dental arch size.
3   Incisal overbite or anterior open bite.
4   Dental arch crowding.

The sources of these variations are:
1   Skeletal factors, in antero-posterior, lateral and vertical dimension.
2   The oral musculature, particularly the tongue.
3   The size of the dentition.
   There is some evidence to support the division of Class 3 occlusions into certain extreme types, but the wide variation of aetiological factors produces many intermediate types which cannot readily be classified.

Treatment objectives include:
1   Reduction of crowding.
2   Correction of reversed overjet.
3   Correction of incisal overbite.
4   Correction of buccal segment relationship, in antero-posterior and lateral dimensions.

The main limiting factors to treatment are the skeletal discrepancy, the size and function of the tongue and the presence of anterior open bite.

Principles of treatment

In the mild Class 3 discrepancy, tipping of upper or lower incisors may be sufficient to correct the reversed overjet, provided sufficient incisal overbite remains for stability.

The more severe Class 3 occlusion may need tipping of both upper and lower anterior segments, or bodily movement of anterior teeth. Vertical relationship of the incisors may need correction with fixed appliances to produce vertical movement.

Unilateral crossbite can be corrected by expansion of the upper arch if mandibular deviation is present. Bilateral crossbites are acceptable if symmetrical, or rapid expansion techniques may be employed.

Treatment with functional appliances in the mixed or early permanent dentition is often used in Class 3 occlusion.

Very severe Class 3 relationships are sometimes beyond the scope of orthodontic treatment alone, and surgical treatment may be indicated.

References

Foster, T. D. & Day, A. J. W. (1974) A survey of malocclusion and the need for orthodontic treatment in a Shropshire school population. *Br J Orthod*, **1**, 73–78.

Haynes, S. (1970) The prevalence of malocclusion in English school children aged 11–12 years. In *Eur Orthod Soc Trans*, pp. 89–98.

Jones, W. B. (1975) A comparison of maxillary basal length in a group of skeletal III cases, with a control group. *Br J Orthod*, **2**, 55–57.

Lewis, A. B. & Roche, A. F. (1988) Late growth changes in the craniofacial skeleton. *Angle Orthod*, **58**, 127–135.

Loh, M. K. & Kerr, W. J. S. (1985) The Function Regulator 111: effects and indications for use. *Br J Orthod*, **12**, 153–157.

Orton, H. S., Sullivan, P. G., Battagel, J. M. & Orton, S. (1983) The management of Class 111 and Class 111 tendency occlusion using headgear to the mandibular dentition. *Br J Orthod*, **10**, 2–12.

Sakamoto, T., Iwase, I., Uka, A. & Nakamura, S. (1984) A roentgenocephalometric study of skeletal changes during and after chin cup treatment. *Am J Orthod*, **85**, 188–189.

Silviera, A. M. (1985) Late mandibular growth during adolescence in the delayed, average and advanced pubertal growth spurt. *Am J Orthod*, **87**, 86–87.

Wendell, P. D. (1984) the effects of chin cup therapy on the mandible: a longitudinal study. *Am J Orthod*, **85**, 188–189 (Abstr.).

19

Orthodontic treatment related to growth

Most orthodontic treatment is carried out on growing children, much of it during the puberal growth period. It is not surprising therefore, that there is increasing interest in the relationship between growth and orthodontic treatment. It seems likely that, in the future, the effects of normal growth will be taken into account to an increasing extent in treatment planning.

The relationship between growth and orthodontics can be examined from four aspects.

1   Normal changes in the dentition and jaws during the growth period.
2   The influence of growth on orthodontic treatment, and the influence of treatment on growth.
3   The assessment of the maximum growth period.
4   The prediction of final form and size of the dento-facial structures.

Normal growth changes in the dentition and jaws

There have been many studies of normal growth changes, both in the size, form and relationships of the dental arches and in the relationship of the jaws. On the whole, most reports have been of mean changes in various populations, and individual variation has been shown to be considerable.

Growth changes in the dental arches

Longitudinal studies of dental arch growth by Van der Linden (1983) and others, have shown that the following mean changes occur:

(a) Dental arch length. After an initial decrease in the primary dentition due to closure of the molar spaces, the dental arch length increases slightly during the eruption of the permanent incisors. Thereafter, the only increase in length is to accommodate the additional permanent molars at the back of the arch, and the length from central incisor to first permanent molar decreases after shedding of the primary molars.

(b) Dental arch width. Little change occurs in the primary dentition. There is an increase in width at the time of eruption of the permanent

incisors, but little or no change from the time of shedding of the primary molars until maturity.

(c) Antero-posterior dental arch relationship. The lower arch shows a slight forward movement in relation to the upper during growth, with a tendency for the incisal overjet to decrease.

(d) Vertical relationship of incisors. There is a tendency for the incisal overbite to decrease slightly in the later stages of growth.

The significance of these findings lies particularly in the fact that the dimensions of the dental arch are established fairly early, and there is a tendency for decrease rather than increase in overall size after the permanent incisors have erupted. Thus it is unrealistic to expect crowding of the teeth to be relieved by dental arch growth. Once established, crowding can usually only be improved by active treatment.

It must be remembered that the above summary of dental arch changes only refers to mean changes. Most investigators stress the wide range of individual variation in growth.

Growth changes in jaw relationships

The results of several growth studies have suggested that the following mean changes occur in the relationships of the jaws during growth.

(a) Profile. The mandible tends to become more prognathic in relation to the maxilla and the base of the skull. The profile therefore, becomes less convex, particularly as forward growth of the nose is proceeding at the same time (Schudy 1974).

(b) Vertical relationship. The progressive increase in the vertical dimension of the jaws usually exhibits a differential between anterior and posterior facial growth. The mean tendency during later adolescent growth is for the vertical development of the mandibular ramus to be predominant, causing an anterior rotation of the mandible and a reduction in the inclination of the mandibular lower border and in the gonial angle (Schudy 1974). Richardson (1971) has pointed out the variation in vertical growth of the anterior segments in patients with anterior open bite, growth of the dento-alveolar elements reducing the open bite in some cases, and predominant increase in facial height maintaining the open bite in others.

(c) Lateral relationship. Growth change in lateral relationship of the jaws is to some extent linked with antero-posterior growth. If forward growth of the mandible is predominant, the divergence of the two sides of the mandibular arch would tend to change the lateral relationship of the upper and lower jaws to each other. There is no evidence, however, for an overall tendency of the lower dental arch to change its lateral relationship with the upper arch during growth, and any change which may occur in the lateral relationship of the jaws is not usually reflected in the tooth relationships.

Perhaps the most important aspect of jaw growth in relation to orthodontic treatment is the apparent tendency of the mandible to develop in a forward and downward direction in relation to the maxilla. If this trend was universal, it would bring a tendency for Class 2 occlusions to improve and Class 3 discrepancies to become more severe, and indeed this sometimes happens. But individual variation occurs in these growth changes as well as in all others. The variation in vertical growth

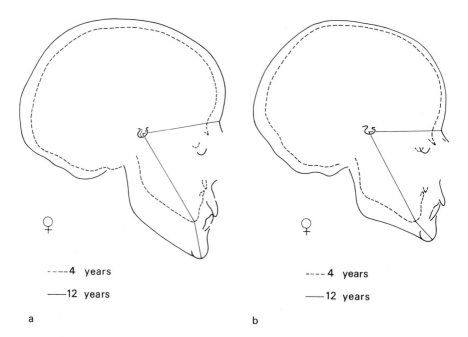

a   b

Fig. 19.1. Superimposed cephalometric tracings of two girls at the ages of 4 years and 12 years, showing variation in amount and direction of facial growth. In (a) growth has been predominantly downward, with backward mandibular rotation. In (b), growth has been predominantly forward, with forward mandibular rotation.

and its variable effect on open bites has been mentioned. Most of the authorities studying growth changes in the jaws have emphasized the extent of variation, not only in the degree of change but also in the direction of differential growth. Thus, in some individuals the mandible may become more retrognathic rather than more prognathic as growth proceeds. Lundström (1969) has pointed out the varying dominance of horizontal growth and vertical growth of the mandible in relation to the maxilla. Bhatia (1971) and Cross (1977) found that in growth changes in mandibular inclination, variation rather than constancy is the general rule (Fig. 19.1). Kerr (1979), reporting a 10-year longitudinal study of facial growth, found that while the mean changes in the relative position of the jaws in the sagittal plane were very small, there was a considerable range of individual variation.

The influence of growth on orthodontic treatment

Tooth movement

It is generally considered that active tooth movement is more readily achieved during periods of growth than it is after growth has ceased. Although there is little objective evidence for this belief, clinical observation suggests that it is correct.

The tissue responses to force applied to the teeth have been studied by Reitan (1951), who observed that response was more rapid in young animals than in those whose growth had been completed. This enhanced response in the growing child, in whom natural changes in bone form and tooth position are taking place, would certainly increase the speed of orthodontic tooth movement. Movement of teeth around the dental arch in the horizontal plane is therefore probably facilitated by normal growth.

Movement in the vertical plane is even more dependent on growth of the jaws, and indeed some movements are unlikely to occur to any great extent after growth has ceased. The reduction of incisal overbite, either with the use of bite planes or of multibanded appliances, depends on the restriction of vertical development of the anterior segments, at the same time allowing vertical development of the buccal segments. For this to be successful, the buccal segments must undergo active vertical growth rather than over-eruption of the teeth. If the dentition is to remain in a stable relationship with the functional musculature, then the overall growth potential must not be exceeded by excessive eruption of the teeth. Such movements in a subject who has finished growing would tend to produce merely over-eruption of the segments and an unstable result.

More localized vertical movements, such as the correction of delayed eruption of individual teeth, are also much more readily and rapidly achieved during the active growth phase.

Relative tooth movement is an important aspect of the relationship between growth and orthodontic treatment. The general direction of developmental movement of the dentition in relation to the skull base is forward and downward. Any orthodontic force applied to individual teeth or groups of teeth in the opposite direction, i.e. backward and upward, has a double effect during the growth phase. The force not only tends to move the teeth, but also restricts the normal forward and downward movement of growth, thereby allowing relative movement of the other dento-alveolar structures. During the period of most rapid jaw growth, it is only necessary to restrict forward movement of a tooth for it to appear to move backward in relation to the other teeth. This relative movement plays an important part in the apparent distal movement of teeth, both with extra-oral traction and with functional appliances (Weinberger 1974; Baumrind *et al.* 1983).

The timing of orthodontic treatment

The state of dental development has often been the main governing factor in the timing of orthodontic treatment. However, dental development is not closely correlated with either chronological age or general developmental age, and in particular is not closely correlated with growth rate. It has been suggested that the timing of orthodontic treatment should be related more to the timing of the various phases of growth than to any other developmental yardstick. As far as active and relative tooth movement is concerned, we have seen that the most rapid growth phase is probably the most favourable time. The most rapid growth phase after infancy is the puberal growth period and many operators utilize this period as far as possible for the main part of corrective orthodontic treatment. Björk (1972) has suggested that four phases of growth lend themselves to different phases of orthodontic treatment. The *infantile period* of most rapid growth is the time for preventive measures. At this stage it is unrealistic to attempt active intervention. The *juvenile period*, when growth rate declines to the pre-puberal minimum, is the time for interceptive measures, such as the correction of local irregularities, particularly those which may cause deviations in the path of closure of the mandible. The *period of most rapid puberal growth* is the time for active corrective treatment, when most tooth movement can be achieved, and this type of treatment will run into the *post-puberal period* in many patients, when growth slows and finally ceases. Until the cessation of growth, tooth positions achieved by active movement may not be stable, and observation or retention may be necessary.

These considerations on tooth movement and the timing of treatment suggest that, in treatment planning, it is often more favourable to assess serial growth records rather than a single 'snapshot' picture of the patient. This is particularly relevant to the assessment of discrepancies in the antero-posterior relationship of the jaws. Serial lateral skull radiographs taken at intervals during the juvenile period would show whether the discrepancy was improving, was stable or was becoming more severe. If *improving* with growth, then functional appliances in the mixed dentition period may be the treatment of choice to take advantage of the natural improvement. If *stable*, then tooth movement would have to be achieved to correct the discrepancy, and this could best be achieved during the puberal growth spurt. If the antero-posterior discrepancy was *becoming more severe* with growth, as sometimes occurs, then even greater tooth movement would be needed, and would need to be continued and maintained until the end of the growth period to avoid the possibility of relapse with growth.

Thus, in some cases, as well as having serial growth records, it is desirable to be able to assess the period of maximum puberal growth, and this will be discussed later in this chapter.

Effect of orthodontic treatment on growth

The concept that orthodontic treatment could influence growth of the jaws, which had been widely held until the advent of cephalometric radiology, gave way to the general principle that orthodontic treatment only affected the position of the dento-alveolar structures. It was felt that, although prolonged forces could influence growing bones, the intensity and duration of the forces used in orthodontic treatment were not sufficient to modify the growth of the basal parts of the jaws. More recently, the idea that growth of the basal structures of the jaws could be influenced by treatment has been revived and investigated.

Two main aspects of orthodontic treatment have been considered. These are the influence of *extra-oral forces* and the effects of *functional appliances*. These two types of treatment can provide the heaviest and the most prolonged forces used in orthodontic therapy, and, in the case of extra-oral force, the anchorage of the force is not dependent on the teeth.

The evidence gained from studies of the effects of these types of treatment on growth has not been consistent.

Extra-oral forces

Several studies have suggested the extra-oral forces applied to retract the maxillary dentition can modify the position of the upper jaw. A number of investigators have produced evidence to show that extra-oral traction can affect the position of the upper jaw during growth, restricting forward development of the maxilla and altering the angulation of the palatal plane. Rindler and Linder Aronson (1980) reported that high-pull extra-oral traction had a permanent effect on the upper anterior face height, while Mills *et al.* (1978) found that similar forces reduced the forward growth of the maxilla without tipping the palatal plane. On the other hand, several investigators have found little or no orthopaedic effect on jaw growth from the use of extra-oral forces (Mills 1978; Baumrind *et al.* 1979), although in a later study Baumrind *et al.* (1983) found that a combination of extra-oral traction and functional appliances did have an orthopaedic effect on maxillary growth.

Functional appliances

Functional appliances have often been considered to produce much of their effect by influencing growth of the jaws. However, there is difference of opinion on this matter. While several studies have failed to find any effects on jaw growth (Calvert 1982; Bolmgren & Moshiri 1986; Hamilton *et al.* 1987), others have reported significant growth effects, particularly on mandibular growth (Dugger 1982; Birkebaek *et al.* 1984; Haynes, 1986). Other aspects of the effects of functional appliances on jaw growth have been discussed in Chapter 15.

Several of the authors of these reports have confirmed that there is considerable individual variation. Furthermore, the studies which show growth changes during treatment have often not been continued to the end of the growth period and it is possible that change induced by treatment may be modified by further growth after treatment is completed. Nevertheless, there is some evidence that slight changes in the position, of the basal elements of the jaws can be produced by heavy extra-oral forces and by some functional appliances, though there is individual variation in response to these forms of treatment. It seems unlikely that orthodontic treatment can overcome the effects of growth where that growth is unfavourable to the attainment of ideals of dento-facial form.

Assessment of the maximal growth period

From the foregoing comments it can be seen that, in some cases there may be advantages in treatment in being able to assess the period of maximum puberal growth. It has been established that, at puberty, the spurt in growth in body height is accompanied by an increased growth rate of the jaws (Hägg & Pancherz 1988). The timing of these phenomena have been investigated in several studies. Ossification of various bones of the hand and wrist has been studied in relation to the puberal growth spurt. Björk and Helm (1967) found a close correlation between the onset of ossification of the adductor sesamoid bone at the metacarpophalyngeal joint of the thumb and the beginning of the maximum growth period. Ossification is said to begin approximately 1 year before the peak of the puberal growth spurt and never occurs after the time of maximum growth. This finding was confirmed by Chapman (1972) who also found that the duration of the growth spurt coincides with the duration of development of the adductor sesamoid, and ends with the onset of fusion of the epiphysis of the proximal phalanx of the thumb, the usual duration being a little over 2 years. Other hand–wrist ossification markers of puberal growth have been reported by Grave and Brown (1976, 1979), by Fishman (1982, 1987) and by Singer (1980), the latter outlining various stages of ossification which compare with stages of growth. Chertkow (1980) has reported not only that the commencement of the growth spurt was closely correlated to the time of certain ossification events in the hand and wrist, but also that there was a high correlation between these events and the stages of mineralization of the lower canine teeth.

On the other hand Houston et al. (1979) and Houston (1980) have found that although the timings of certain ossification events are related to the puberal growth spurt, there is considerable uncertainty in the prediction of timing of the growth spurt in individuals, which makes the use of hand–wrist radiographs of limited value for this purpose. Chmura (1984) reported that ossification of the ulnar sesamoid was not found to predict the onset, duration or rate of the puberal growth spurt.

The age of menarche in girls is also considered to be related to the puberal growth spurt. Björk and Helm (1967) have found that menarche occurred some 17 months after the peak of puberal growth and never before the time of maximum growth. This finding was confirmed by Dermaut and O'Reilly (1978) in relation to vertical growth of the face, although O'Reilly (1979) again emphasized the individual variation in the timing of growth of maxillary length, maximum growth sometimes occurring before, and sometimes after menarche.

A different method of determination of the maximum growth period has been proposed by Sullivan (1983). It is based on consecutive measurements of standing height to determine changes in growth velocity, from which a prediction of the time of maximum velocity is made. Again, individual variation limits the clinical value of this method.

The completion of mandibular growth coincides with the completion of growth in body height, which can be assessed by radiographic examination of the radius at the wrist. The radial epiphysis normally fuses at or slightly before the stage of completion of skeletal growth. As previously mentioned, growth of the mandible tends to go on somewhat longer than growth in other parts of the face.

Thus, while radiographic examination of the hand and wrist, serial height measurements and the age of menarche might give some guidance to the period of maximum growth and to the final completion of growth, in clinical orthodontics individual variation seems likely to make this information of limited value.

The prediction of final form and size of the dento-facial structures

It would often be of value, in planning and carrying out orthodontic treatment, to be able to predict the final form and size of the face and jaws after growth has ceased. If this were possible, the objectives of treatment could be more realistic. The effects of growth could be harnessed in modifying final tooth positions and attempts to achieve impossible tooth positions could be avoided.

The prediction of skeletal height has been well documented (Tanner 1981). It depends essentially on population studies to determine the relationship between height at given ages and final height. Individual variation reduces the accuracy of prediction, and it is only possible to predict the height range at quoted probability levels. The prediction of facial form is more complex and inevitably less accurate. Skeletal height is a single measurement of the total increments of the growth of various bones. Facial form has many parameters, each of which is only predictable within certain limits of accuracy. Taken all together to give a final face, the limits of accuracy must be fairly wide. Nevertheless several methods of prediction have been proposed. These methods involve first the definition of certain key parameters of the face, usually assessed on standardized skull radiographs. Mean growth increments are applied to these dimensions, the means being derived from population studies. Finally a prediction of final overall form is built up from the estimated increments on the key parameters.

These systems of prediction have received support from some authors (Schulhof *et al.* 1977; Thames *et al.* 1985) and are probably satisfactory for many patients whose growth changes differ little from the population means. There are, however, the two main problems in their use, apart from the possibility of measurement errors, which limit all forecasts on growth and development. These are the problem of defining the population from which the mean values are derived and the problem of the extent of individual variation from the means. The mean values of one population are not necessarily applicable to patients in another country, or even in another part of the same country. Many authorities are of the opinion that, because of these difficulties, current methods of growth prediction are of only limited value (Greenberg & Johnston 1975; Houston 1979).

Summary

Studies of growth and development have outlined mean changes in dental arch and jaw form, size and relationship, but there is considerable individual variation.

It would seem that the modifications of growth that can be brought about by orthodontic treatment are likely to be confined to a large extent to the dento-alveolar structures, with only minor modifications being possible in the form and relationships of the jaws.

A knowledge of growth trends gained from serial records would be of value in determining the general type and direction of growth changes in many cases. If active treatment is to be instituted, tooth movement is likely to be easier during the puberal growth period, the pre-puberal period being the optimum time for interceptive measures. During the post-puberal period until growth ceases, further natural change in tooth position may occur, and it may be necessary to apply retention through this period.

The prediction of growth changes in size, form and relationship of the jaws is uncertain, due to individual variation, though it is probably useful in those patients who do not deviate markedly from the population means.

References

Baumrind, S., Korn, E. L., Isaacson, R. J., West, E. E. & Molthen, R. (1983) Quantitative analysis of the orthodontic and orthopaedic effects of maxillary traction. *Am J Orthod,* **84**, 384–398.

Baumrind, S., Molthen, R., West, E. E. & Miller, D. M. (1979). Distal displacement of the maxilla and the upper first molar. *Am J Orthod,* **75**, 630–640.

Bhatia, S. N. (1971) A longitudinal study of the SN–mandibular, Frankfort–mandibular plane angles. *Dent Practit,* **21**, 285–289.

Birkebaek, L., Melsen, B. & Terps, S. (1984) A laminagraphic study of the alterations in the Temporo-Mandibular joint following activator treatment. *Eur J Orthod,* **6**, 257–266.

Björk, A. (1972) Timing of interceptive orthodontic measures based on stages of maturation. *Eur Orthod Soc Trans,* 61–74.

Björk, A. & Helm, S. (1967) Prediction of the age of maximum puberal growth in body height. *Angle Orthod,* **37**, 134–143.

Bolmgren, G. A. & Moshiri, F. (1986) Bionator treatment in Class II Division I. *Angle Orthod,* **56**, 255–262.

Calvert, F. J. (1982) An assessment of Andresen therapy on Class II Division I malocclusion. *Br J Orthod,* **9**, 149–153.

Chapman, S. M. (1972) Ossification of the adductor sesamoid and the adolescent growth spurt. *Angle Orthod,* **42**, 236–244.

Chertkow, S. (1980) Tooth mineralisation as an indicator of the pubertal growth spurt. *Am J Orthod,* **77**, 79–81.

Chmura, L. (1984) Relationship between sesamoid calcification and facial growth. *J Dent Res,* **63**, 163.

Cross, J. J. (1977) Facial growth: before, during and following orthodontic treatment. *Am J Orthod,* **71**, 68–78.

Dermaut, C. R. & O'Reilly, M. I. T. (1978) Changes in anterior facial height in girls during puberty. *Angle Orthod,* **48**, 163–171.

Dugger, G. C. (1982) Orofacial change resulting from Fränkel appliance treatment. *Am J Orthod,* **82**, 354. Abstract.

Fishman, L. S. (1982) Radiographic evaluation of skeletal maturation. *Angle Orthod,* **52**, 88–112.

Fishman, L. (1987) Maturational patterns and prediction during adolescence. *Angle Orthod,* **57**, 178–193.

Gilda, J. E. (1974) Analysis of linear facial growth. *Angle Orthod,* **44**, 1–14. *J Orthod,* **69**, 611–619.

Grave, K. C. & Brown, T. (1979) Carpal radiographs in orthodontic treatment. *Am J Orthod,* **75**, 27–45.

Greenberg, L. Z. & Johnston, L. E. (1975) Computerised prediction: the accuracy of a contemporary long range forecast. *Am J Orthod,* **67**, 243–252.

Hägg, U. & Pancherz, H. (1988) Dentofacial orthopaedics in relation to chronological age, growth period and skeletal development. *Eur J Orthod,* **10**, 169–176.

Hamilton, S. D., Sinclair, P. M. & Hamilton, R. H. (1987) A cephalometric, tomographic and dental cast evaluation of Fränkel therapy. *Am J Orthod,* **92**, 427–434.

Haynes, S. (1986) A cephalometric study of mandibular changes in modified function regulator (Fränkel) treatment. *Am J Orthod*, **90**, 308–320.

Houston, W. J. B. (1979) The current status of facial growth prediction: a review. *Br J Orthod*, **6**, 11–17.

Houston, W. J. B. (1980) Relationships between skeletal maturity estimated from hand–wrist radiographs and the timing of the adolescent growth spurt. *Eur J Orthod*, **2**, 81–93.

Houston, W. J. B., Miller, J. C. & Tanner, J. M. (1979) Prediction of the timing of the adolescent growth spurt from ossification events in hand–wrist films. *Br J Orthod*, **6**, 145–152.

Kerr, W. J. S. (1979) A longitudinal cephalometric study of dentofacial growth from 5 to 15 years. *Br J Orthod*, **6**, 115–121.

Lundström, A. (1969) Horizontal and vertical growth of the incision superior, incision inferior and Menton. *Europ Orthod Soc Trans*, 125–136.

Mills, J. R. E. (1978) The effect of orthodontic treatment on the skeletal pattern. *Brit J Orthod*, **5**, 133–143.

Mills, C. M., Holman, R. G. & Graber, T. M. (1978) Heavy intermittent cervical traction in Class II treatment: A longitudinal cephalometric assessment. *Am J Orthod*, **74**, 361–379.

O'Reilly, M. T. (1979) A longitudinal growth study: maxillary length at puberty in females. *Angle Orthod*, **49**, 234–238.

Reitan, K. (1951) The initial tissue reaction incident to orthodontic tooth movement. *Acta Odont Scand*, **9**, Suppl. 6.

Richardson, A. (1971) Facial growth and the prognosis for anterior open bite—a longitudinal study. *Eur Orthod Soc Trans*, 149–157.

Rindler, A. & Linder-Aronson, S. (1980) The long-term effect of high pull headgear on the incisor region of the maxilla. *Eur J Orthod*, **2**, 105–111.

Schulhof, R. J., Nakamura, S. & Williamson, W. V. (1977) Prediction of abnormal growth in Class III malocclusions. *Am J Orthod*, **71**, 421–430.

Schudy, G. F. (1974) Post-treatment craniofacial growth: Its implications in orthodontic treatment. *Am J Orthod*, **65**, 39–57.

Singer, J. (1980) Physiologic timing of orthodontic treatment. *Angle Orthod*, **50**, 322–333.

Sullivan, P. G. (1983) Prediction of the pubertal growth spurt by measurement of standing height. *Eur J Orthod*, **5**, 189–196.

Tanner, J. M. (1981) *A History of the Study of Human Growth.* Cambridge, Cambridge University Press.

Thames, T.L., Sinclair, P. M. & Alexander, R. G. (1985) The accuracy of computerised growth prediction in Class II high-angle cases. *Am J Orthod*, **87**, 398–405.

Van der Linden, F. P. G. M. (1983) *Development of the Dentition.* Chicago, Quintessence Publishing Co.

Weinberger, T. W. (1974) Extra-oral traction and functional appliances—a cephalometric comparison. *Br J Orthod*, **1**, 35–39.

20

Orthodontics and preventive dentistry

The prevention of dental disease is one of the most important aspects of dental care. Orthodontics can be related to prevention in three ways:

1 The prevention of malocclusion.
2 The role of orthodontic treatment in the prevention of other dental diseases.
3 The prevention of dental disease during orthodontic treatment.

The prevention of malocclusion

We have seen in earlier chapters that, on the whole, the main aetiological factors in malocclusion seem to be inherited. The skeletal pattern of the jaws, the form of the oral musculature and the size of the dentition are all governed largely by genetic factors. Most of the localized factors, such as supernumerary teeth and hypodontia, probably have an inherited background. *Primary prevention* or modification of these features is therefore hardly possible. Even those few aetiological factors which are the result of the environment, such as trauma, are not really preventable, with the exception of early loss of primary teeth. Early loss of teeth could be prevented, but we have seen that this is not a primary cause of malocclusion, but merely aggravates crowding problems in certain conditions. Primary prevention of malocclusion by modification of its aetiological factors is therefore not practicable in most patients, in the present state of knowledge. There is always likely to be the need for corrective treatment.

Secondary prevention is, however, of practical importance in orthodontics. Two aspects of secondary prevention can be outlined.

(a) The prevention of the basic aetiological features producing their maximum adverse effect. This applies mostly to the localized factors, and can be illustrated with reference to the tuberculate supernumerary tooth. If such a tooth is left in place for several years, the eruption of the permanent upper central incisor is delayed. The adjacent teeth are likely to encroach on the space, and a much more severe occlusal problem results, which could have been prevented by removing the supernumerary tooth earlier.

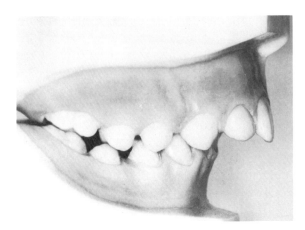

Fig. 20.1. The early extraction of the first permanent molars has allowed the second molars to move forward during eruption, thus closing the spaces and making correction of the Class 2 occlusion more difficult.

(b) The prevention of factors which make an established malocclusion more difficult to correct. Perhaps the prime example of this is the illtimed extraction of teeth. Fig. 20.1 shows a Class 2 Division 1 occlusion in which treatment has been made more difficult by removal of the upper first permanent molars, allowing the second molars to move forward into the spaces.

Thus, while primary prevention of malocclusion is unrealistic, secondary prevention can help to avoid malocclusion or reduce the need for treatment in some cases. The key to prevention of this kind is awareness. The early assessment of the child, followed by regular review, and treatment at the appropriate time if necessary, will do much to reduce malocclusion to the basic non-preventable level.

Orthodontic treatment in the prevention of dental disease

While it may seem logical to assume that the correction of malocclusion plays an important part in the prevention of other dental disease, there is some difference of opinion and little strong evidence on this matter. If malocclusion is related to periodontal disease and dental caries, then orthodontic treatment should be beneficial in preventing these widespread dental diseases. Studies of the relationship between occlusal factors and dental and periodontal disease have, however, produced some conflicting results.

With regard to periodontal disease, while several earlier investigators failed to find any consistent relationship between malocclusion and periodontal disease, a number of more recent studies have reported low but statistically significant correlations between irregularity of the teeth and dental plaque, gingivitis and calculus. (Behlfelt *et al.* 1981; Buckley 1981; El Mangoury *et al.* 1987; Addy *et al.* 1988). On the other hand Polson *et al.* (1988) found no significant difference in any of the periodontal variables in a group of patients 10 years after orthodontic treatment when compared with a similar group with untreated mal-occlusion, and Shefter and Fall (1984) also found that occlusal features seemed to play a minimal role in the progress of periodontal disease. Similarly, Helm *et al.* (1984) found that untreated malocclusion did not seem to predispose to tooth loss in the adult.

There is little evidence on the relationship between dental caries prevalence and malocclusion, though a survey of a large sample of schoolchildren in England and Wales found significantly more dental caries and gingival inflammation in children with crowded dentitions (Todd 1975).

It is difficult to strike a balance between these somewhat conflict-ing reports. A consensus, together with clinical experience, suggests that there is some relationship between certain occlusal discrepancies and periodontal disease, and possibly dental caries. If a necessary feature in the aetiology of these diseases is dental plaque, it would seem reasonable to believe that any occlusal condition which predisposes to the accumulation of dental plaque, particularly by making natural or artificial cleansing of the teeth more difficult, may be related to periodontal disease. Severe crowding and irregularity of the teeth may constitute such a condition. In addition, any direct occlusal trauma to the gingival tissues, such as may sometimes be seen with excessive incisal overbite, may cause gingival disease, as may trauma resulting from premature occlusal contacts.

It can be concluded, therefore, that orthodontic treatment has some part to play in the prevention of the main dental diseases, even though ideal dental occlusion is not always a pre-requisite for a healthy mouth.

There is even less evidence on the role of orthodontic treatment in the prevention of functional disorders of the masticatory apparatus. While it appears reasonable to believe that a well aligned and functionally well related dentition is important in the prevention of functional disorders, Helm *et al.* (1984), studying 30-year-old adults, reported that untreated malocclusion did not seem to predispose to such problems. Further investigation is needed on this aspect of the subject.

The prevention of dental disease during orthodontic treatment

Active orthodontic treatment involves the wearing of appliances. Any appliance worn in the mouth, no matter how carefully designed and fitted, has potential for producing dental and periodontal disease. Hollender *et al.* (1980) and Hamp *et al.* (1982) reported that the use of fixed appliances produced a slight but significant irreversible loss of periodontal support, although Huber *et al.* (1987) found that this problem could be minimized by regular monthly prophylaxis and oral hygiene instruction. O'Reilly and Featherstone (1987) and Øgaard *et al.* (1988) have also reported early demineralization of teeth in relation to fixed appliances, and again found that such development could be inhibited or reversed by the use of topical fluorides.

It is of considerable importance that orthodontic treatment benefits the patient by correcting occlusal faults and does not produce adverse effects on the patient by increasing other dental disease problems. A planned programme of preventive care is therefore necessary for all patients who are to have appliance treatment. Such a programme can be outlined as follows.

Before treatment begins

The dental condition should be as good as possible before orthodontic treatment is started. Dental caries and periodontal disease should be treated as far as possible, consistent with any limitations imposed by the malocclusion. The patient should be given careful instruction in home care, particularly with regard to oral hygiene and diet, and must be willing and able to maintain an adequate standard of home care. A poor initial dental condition does not necessarily mean that orthodontic treatment should not be applied, but good patient co-operation and optimum dental health must be achieved if treatment is to be successful.

At the beginning of treatment

Immediately before fitting any appliance the teeth should be cleaned and polished. Topical fluoride may be applied unless direct bonding is planned. In some circumstances newly erupted, caries-free posterior teeth may benefit from the application of fissure sealant before the topical fluoride application.

Careful instruction should be given regarding the hygiene of the appliance. With removable appliances there is a tendency to develop candida infections if appliance hygiene is poor. This results in acute hypertrophic stomatitis, with swelling and redness of the gingival and mucosal tissue under the appliance, sometimes associated with angular cheilitis (Fig. 20.2). In this condition, the organisms can be isolated mainly on the plaque covering the fitting surface of the appliance rather than on the mucosal tissue (Davenport 1970). Specific medication may be necessary to treat the condition, but its prevention can be achieved by adequate oral and appliance hygiene.

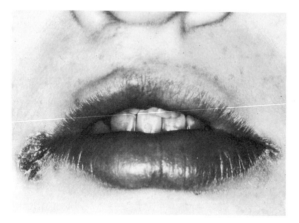

a

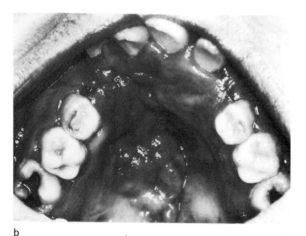

b

Fig. 20.2. Angular cheilitis and hypertrophic stomatitis associated with *Candida* infection, the result of poor appliance hygiene.

During treatment

There are two aspects of preventive care during orthodontic appliance treatment, these being the maintenance of oral health and the application of regular topical fluorides to the teeth. At each visit of the patient, apart from checking the progress of treatment and carrying out any necessary work on the appliance, the general state of oral health should be assessed. This is particularly important in relation to oral hygiene. Disclosing solutions may be used to demonstrate dental plaque, and continuing instruction in oral hygiene is often necessary. It need hardly be said that all necessary operative treatment should be continued.

Regular applications of fluoride to the teeth are likely to be beneficial, particularly during prolonged courses of appliance treatment. Øgaard et al. (1988) have found that a regime of topical application of acidulated phosphate fluoride with 0.6% F at pH 1.9 at each monthly visit inhibited the development of decalcified lesions in patients wearing fixed orthodontic appliances, while Geiger et al. (1988) recommended the application of 1.2% F at pH 3.2 immediately after bonding, plus daily rinsing with 0.05% sodium fluoride solution. The daily use of a fluoride toothpaste or gel is also recommended.

With the use of methods such as those outlined above, before and during treatment, there is no reason why orthodontic treatment should bring any permanent hazard to the oral health of the patient. Orthodontic treatment, carefully planned and carried out, should be and can be completely beneficial to the patient in correcting occlusal faults which have adverse effects on function, oral health and appearance.

References

Addy, M., Griffiths, G. S., Dummer, P. M. H., Kingdon, A., Hicks, R., Hunter, M. L., Newcombe, R. G. & Shaw, W. C. (1988) The association between tooth irregularity and plaque accumulation, gingivitis and caries in 11–12 year old children. *Eur J Orthod*, **10**, 76–83.

Behlfelt, K., Ericsson, L., Jacobson, L. & Linder–Aronson, S. (1981) The occurrence of plaque and gingivitis and its relationship to tooth alignment within the dental arches. *J Clin Periodontol*, **8**, 329–337.

Buckley, L. A. (1981) The relationship between malocclusion, gingival inflammation, plaque and calculus. *J Periodontol*, **52**, 35–40.

El-Mangoury, N. H., Gaarfar, S. M. & Mostafa, Y. A. (1987) Mandibular anterior crowding and periodontal disease. *Angle Orthod*, **57**, 33–38.

Geiger, A. M., Gorelick, L., Gwinnett, A. J. & Griswold, P. G. (1988) The effect of a fluoride programme on white spot formation during orthodontic treatment. *Am J Orthod*, **93**, 29–37.

Hamp, S. E., Lundström, F. & Nyman, S. (1982) Periodontal conditions in adolescents subjected to multiband orthodontic treatment with controlled oral hygiene. *Eur J Orthod*, **4**, 77–86.

Helm, S., Kreiborg, S. & Solow, B. (1984) Malocclusion at adolescence related to self-reported tooth loss and functional disorders in adulthood. *Am J Orthod*, **85**, 393–400.

Hollender, L., Ronnerman, A. & Thilander, B. (1980) Root resorption, marginal bone support and clinical crown length in orthodontically treated patients. *Eur J Orthod*, **2**, 197–205.

Huber, S. J., Vernino, A. R. & Nanda, R. S. (1987) Professional prophylaxis and its effect on the periodontium of full-banded orthodontic patients. *Am J Orthod*, **91**, 321–327.

Øgaard, B., Rølla, G. & Arends, J. (1988) Orthodontic appliances and enamel demineralisation. *Am J Orthod*, **94**, 68–73.

O'Reilly, M. M. & Featherstone, J. D. B. (1987) Demineralisation and remineralisation around orthodontic appliances: an *in vivo* study. *Am J Orthod*, **92**, 33–40.

Polson, A. M., Subtelny, J. D., Meitner, S. W., Polson, A. P., Sommers, E. W., Iker, H. P. & Reed B. E. (1988) Long-term periodontal status after orthodontic treatment. *Am J Orthod*, **93**, 51–58.

Shefter, G. J. & Fall, W. T. (1984) Occlusal relations and periodontal status in human adults. *J Periodontol*, **55**, 368–375.

Todd, J. E. (1975) *Children's Dental Health in England and Wales, 1973*. London, HMSO.

Index